In the Failing Light

In the Failing Light

A MEMOIR

❧

DAVID TILLMAN

CREATIVE ARTS BOOK COMPANY

Berkeley • California 1999

In the Failing Light is published by Donald S. Ellis
and distributed by Creative Arts Book Company.

For information contact:
Creative Arts Book Company
833 Bancroft Way
Berkeley, California 94710

ISBN 088739-177x
Library of Congress Catalog Number 98-71381

Printed in the United States of America

In the Failing Light

Chapter 1

*"S*HE'LL GROW UP WITH NO MEMORY OF ME," my wife remarked, staring sadly at the infant seated on my lap.

"She'll remember you," I promised as I gazed idly at the blood pressure cuff dangling from the pale wall. "You're going to live to be a hundred."

"No," she protested. "I won't live to see Christmas."

I reached over and patted her knee. "You'll be fine."

"I'm going to die," she sighed. "I'll never see our daughter grow up." She stared again at the nine-month-old girl, and forced a weak smile.

It was our third wedding anniversary, and we were spending the morning in the examination room of a local surgeon.

"I'll do a biopsy, anyway," he explained. "But it's obviously advanced breast cancer."

"Will you have to cut me?" my wife asked anxiously.

"For the biopsy, yes," he answered gently. "No mastectomy, though. It's too late."

"Then I'm going to die."

Perhaps not, he told us. Not with tamoxifen. He had one patient taking tamoxifen who was still alive after ten years.

"No. I'm going to die," she replied with quiet resignation.

"How could they have missed the cancer?" I asked, fighting back my anger as I stood before her in our bedroom.

"They missed it," she replied calmly from the bed, where she sat knitting me a sweater.

"But you were over forty, and you were having your first baby, and they watched you so closely," I continued, feeling the hot flush of my cheeks. "How could they have missed it?"

"They missed it." She set her knitting aside and patted the bed.

I sat down beside her, a feeling of calm returning as our bodies touched. "And you wanted to nurse your baby, but your nipple was sucked inside-out by the cancer. How did they miss that?"

"They did."

"And you even had a mammogram," I said.

"Those miss it all the time," she replied.

We walked across the scattered weeds and rocks of the small park that bordered our yard, and the memory of the doctor visit followed us.

"You heard him," she said. "They caught it too late."

"No," I argued as I walked beside her with our golden retriever tugging ahead on her leash. "You're going to live to be a hundred."

A dog ran across the field, barking. It attacked our dog as I held on to her leash.

"You should keep him tied," I remarked as the owner trotted over.

"I've seen your dog loose chasing birds," he replied defensively.

"Yes, but she didn't attack you."

"Fuck off," he snapped.

Fuck off.

We've got cancer. Fuck off to that. Fuck off to crime, and hunger, and a lot of other things. Don't fuck off to a small family walking sadly across a field of stones.

"I want to go away," my wife cried.

Flee. Yes, flee. The three of us, to some distant corner of the globe where cancer can't find us.

"For the weekend," she added.

"For just the weekend?" I asked.

"Yes. Can we do that?"

Sure. A weekend. A week. A month. A year. Eternity. It no longer mattered. What we had was gone. The world still looked the same, but something was gone from it. All that was left was so fragile: my wife, my baby daughter.

"Have you ever been to Lake George?"

"No," she replied. "Is it pretty?"

"It was," I said. "But that was thirty years ago."

We were silent as we approached the lake. Distant thunderclouds hung low over the region.

"Is it always stormy here?" she asked anxiously.

"In the summer," I explained. "Hot air, cold air, all these lakes and rivers."

"But it's sunny, too?"

"Yes," I replied. "After the storms have passed."

"It's not a very pretty town," she observed, staring out the side window as I steered our car through the holiday traffic.

Wax museums, T-shirt shops, wooden Indians. Roller coasters!

"No, but the lake is pretty."

"It's too bad the town comes before the lake," she sighed. "First impressions."

"And last impressions, too, when we leave."

"Couldn't we go home a different way?" she asked. "What's north?"

"Vermont, I think."

"No," she replied. "Vermont is east."

"Northeast," I corrected her.

We walked among the ruins of a faded estate. A part of it had been sold as condos, but the rest was slowly disappearing into the woods.

Deep in the woods, in the middle of a small clearing, a crumpled arch marked the entrance to a little garden. The fountain was full of leaves, and the stone dolphin that had at one time spouted water had dropped onto the cracked mosaic patio and split in half.

"It's a strange place for a garden," she observed.

"I suppose these woods were lawns back then," I surmised.

"It's a sad place," she said. "Do you know any place happy?"

"The game farm," I replied.

"A zoo?"

"No," I said. "It's better than a zoo. It's a game farm, and the animals run free."

But it was a zoo. My childhood memories had tricked me. And the vast fields that the animals had pranced across when I was five were actually cages now that I saw them again with my adult eyes.

A rhino was trapped on an island the size of a two car garage.

We watched sadly as he trotted round and round, wearing a path into the ground that was six inches lower than the surrounding land.

"Let's see the bear show," I suggested.

"Like Clark's Trading Post?" she asked hopefully. "He loved his bears. You could see that."

"This is just like Clark's Trading Post."

Large groups of children sat on bleachers, laughing at the bears. Adults, too. I looked over to see if she was laughing, but she was crying.

"You're safe here," I said gently. "Don't think about what the doctor said."

"I'm not crying for me," she said, pointing. "I'm crying for the bears."

The humiliation. Wild creatures stuffed into pink tutus, riding about on undersized tricycles. Youngsters jeering, throwing popcorn. It wasn't like Clark's. They didn't love their bears here.

I cried, too, but I cried for my wife.

We visited a reproduction fort in town that sold plastic tomahawks. Made in Taiwan. Lacquer-coated photos of leaping trout pasted to the front of cedar slabs said 'Welcome To Lake George.' Plastic hula skirts!

"Let's go home," she said.

"Don't you want a ride on the lake first?" I asked.

"No. It might disappoint me," she sighed. "We'll drive north and I'll see the lake from a safe distance."

"Through Vermont," I said.

"That would be east," she replied with a smile. "Not north."

"Northeast." I smiled back.

To Fort Ticonderoga. The Green Mountain Boys. Ethan Allen before he sold furniture. No plastic tomahawks. Quality! We had to stop.

"Look! The family pants." She grinned as she stood before a glass case on the second floor of the historic fort's museum, in the rebuilt officer's barracks.

There they were. They looked just like them—the family pants. Ten generations ago, more or less, my family fought with the British in the French and Indian War. A generation later, we changed sides and fought against the British in the Revolutionary War. The family pants were what remained of those distant conflicts. Originally, there were more than pants: an officer's jacket, a cartridge belt, a sword, a musket. There had been a powder horn; I'd seen that at my grandfather's farm when I was young. Each generation split the heirlooms among their sons, breaking up the set further and further until all that remained for me were the family pants, with blood and a bullet hole in the backside.

Run away. That's what my ancestor had done. Shot in the backside. Run fast, run far, run from danger. You can see it in the pants. It's in my genes. Come, my little family, let us run now from the danger that haunts us.

"Oh, look at that picture," she said. "Why did they do that?"

It was the fort, before reconstruction. Gnarled trees grew from the remnants of the eroding battlements. There were gaping holes and crumbling towers where after the war, the local farmers had pilfered the black stone to build their barns.

We could see by the very darkness that it was a haunted place then. But the dark spirits were now replaced by smiling tourists.

"It wasn't historic back then," I said. "It was an abandoned fort with a good supply of stone."

"I suppose so," she said. "It would be like taking cinder blocks from an abandoned Wal-Mart."

Except Wal-Marts are never abandoned.

We returned home to find that nothing had changed. We

could have circled the globe a hundred times. We could have driven on and on, turning down nameless roads that appeared on no maps, kept going and never stopped, but our troubles would still have been with us.

There was no hiding from cancer.

Chapter 2

I SENT MY WIFE AWAY. And my child. For a month she stayed with her sister in the suburbs of Boston, and I stayed behind in a house that we no longer thought of as ours. I was a trespasser.

"I'm dying," she said. It was her last day at our old home. Ever. I held her door open as she climbed into our car. "I'm dying, aren't I?"

"Ignore what that doctor said," I replied angrily. "He was a jerk."

He was a jerk. He was upset when the first tests came back and showed no cancer in her bones.

"I can tell by her skin color," he had proclaimed. "She's got cancer in her bones and liver!" But he was wrong about the bones. Nobody can see cancer by your skin color. Go down to the local hardware store and check your arm against the paint samples? If only diagnoses were as easy as that.

"It's in her liver, though. I was right about the liver!" the doctor had shouted jubilantly when the second set of test results came back.

I hadn't hung up the phone yet, but the decision was already made. Send her to Boston. Find a real doctor. What sort of oncologist sets up practice in the sparsely populated woods of northeastern Connecticut anyway? What sort of doctor cheers when he finds cancer?

"Don't listen to that jerk," I cautioned my wife.

She smiled sadly at our daughter sitting safely in a baby carrier, strapped in the car's back seat with a pile of soft stuffed animals.

"You'll live to be a hundred."

She wanted to go to Boston, to be near her family, to die near her family. I wanted her to go to Boston, to find a better doctor, to live near her family. To live to be a hundred.

She stayed with her sister in a house that was full before she got there.

"It's crowded," she said, her voice sounding far-off as she spoke to me through the telephone. "They don't complain, but we're crowding them."

"I'll rent you a house," I replied.

"With a back yard?"

"And a tree," I promised. "We've never had a real tree before."

"And a shady spot to set our hammock," she sighed. "That would be nice."

I found a house, a raised ranch. It had a big back yard. The house was next to the railroad tracks, though. Not just next to the railroad tracks—it was where the tracks crossed the road, and the freight trains had to blast their horns at two A.M. so that people sneaking their cars around the crossing gates would spend their final moments terrified out of their wits by the sound of impending doom.

I stayed behind, living alone in our old house. It was no longer a home. My in-laws had come and taken most of our stuff to Boston so that my wife could be surrounded by all her things.

What remained was a mattress and a portable television. One plate, a fork, and a knife. A toothbrush, an electric shaver, and five pairs of underpants—jockey shorts with the elastics growing weak. Some shirts and pants, and a frying pan.

Even our dog was gone, sent away to live with strangers.

It was Wednesday evening and I couldn't stand the loneliness any longer, so I hopped in my Daytona and drove two hours to the rented house.

"What happened to your hair?" I asked. I hid behind a bouquet of flowers as she opened the front door. She didn't expect me until Friday. Surprise!

"What are you doing here?" she asked.

"I missed you," I replied. "What happened to your hair?"

I stepped into the rented house and set the flowers on the staircase. Her head was wrapped tight in a red checkered bandanna, like she had been baking.

"I cut it off," she explained.

"I'm sorry."

"I couldn't stand watching clumps of it falling off into my lap," she said sadly. "So I cut it all off."

Adriamycin. 5-FU. Poison the body, kill the cancer, and hope that the patient lives.

Hair falling out—it was good, and it was bad. Bad because

every morning, she looked in the mirror and saw, yes, she had cancer. Good because it meant something was happening. If hair cells were dying, cancer cells were dying.

She started to cry.

"But I still love you," I said.

"No, you can't," she sobbed. "One breast is a tight little knot, and the hormones have made me fat. And now I have no hair."

"But I do still love you," I vowed. I watched as more tears welled up in her eyes. But the earlier tears of sadness were washed away now by tears of sullen happiness, tears of subtle love.

I slipped my arms around her waist. We embraced there on the front landing of the rented house, and I couldn't let her go. The face of a happy infant appeared at the top of the staircase, and I smiled up at her.

"How's my little pumpkin been?" I asked.

"Good," my wife replied. "My sister took her most of the day so I could rest."

We climbed the stairs to the living room. I scooped up my daughter and carried her to the center of the room, where I set her down on the pink carpeting. I sat down beside the little girl, and my wife sat on the sofa where she always sat, where she could look out and see the cars go by, carrying people with normal lives off to their daily activities. She picked up a medical book she had been reading and flipped it open.

"She's going to grow up and not remember anything about me." My wife looked up from the medical book, and I could see the tears in her eyes again. She looked lovingly at the child who played beside me on the pink carpeting. "That's the hardest part."

"You won't die," I replied firmly.

"You'll tell her about me, won't you?" She set the medical

book aside. She had read it over and over, but nothing in it ever changed.

"Don't read it anymore." I had told her that many times. "They're wrong. You'll live to be a hundred."

She sighed and forced a smile. "Did we sell the house?" she asked, turning her attention outside. Summer. Her favorite time of year, but now she was too sick to enjoy it.

"No," I replied. "The real estate agent says we'll have to drop the price some more."

"Did you?"

Did I? Could I? Fifty thousand dollars already sunk in the place and the real estate agent was telling me it was all gone. Poof.

"No," I said. "But I finally told my boss that you were sick."

"You shouldn't have." She continued staring out the window as though the concerns of the living were no longer hers.

"I did."

"Did he fire you?"

"No," I replied. "He told me to stay as long as I could, to leave when I needed to. 'Don't worry about giving two weeks notice,' he said. 'Take care of your wife.'"

"That doesn't sound like IBM," she said.

"It makes me sorry to leave," I replied. "But I found a job in Boston. They called me today with an offer."

My wife smiled weakly. She didn't ask how much it paid. It paid half of what I had been making. That was okay. A mortgage on the house, a rental condo losing money, rent on another house, medical bills, a car payment. When your feet no longer touch the bottom, does it matter how deep the water gets?

"Then you'll be moving up here?" she asked hopefully.

"The end of the month," I replied.

"Two weeks," she said.

That was all. Two weeks.

Chapter 3

❧

MY NEW JOB STARTED as summer came to an end. By then the city had taken on the ripe aroma of a long season of heat and decay, of the nearby sea, of the sweaty feet of a million passing tourists.

I worked in the investment field for a company that picked stocks for their clients. What they really did was show the computer how to throw random darts at the *Wall Street Journal*, wrap it up in a mysterious veneer of investment jargon, and call it science.

The pay was okay. It paid the bills—the Boston bills, but not the Connecticut bills.

"I'm trying to sell the Connecticut house," I told the bank that held our mortgage. They knew real estate, and they knew it would be a hard sell, but they were patient and left us alone.

"I'm trying to sell the condo," I told the second bank, the

one that held the mortgage on the condo. I couldn't sell the condo in 1987 and had rented it out at a loss for four years. The market would improve, I thought, but it didn't.

They knew real estate, the second bank. They knew no one could sell a condo in 1991 any better than they could in 1987, but they didn't care.

"I can pay you seven hundred a month now, but I'll have to owe you the other two hundred," I explained to the loan officer.

"You have to pay it all," he replied curtly.

"I can't."

"We're going to sue you then." You and your sick wife and your young child.

That bank went under along with us. Sometimes there is justice. I'd like to think that I was the one that brought them down. That would make a lot of things right.

On October 4, 1991, we filed for bankruptcy. That's a date I'll always remember. Wedding anniversary, child's birthday, bankruptcy filing.

"Try suing us now, bank!"

"No, thank you. We'll just go under along with you."

Justice.

I filled out the paperwork myself and brought it to the bankruptcy court in person.

"You're a lawyer," the clerk remarked as she leafed through the paperwork.

"No," I replied. "I'm a bankrupt."

"But your paperwork is much better than most lawyers." She smiled. Calling me a lawyer wasn't meant to be an insult.

I smiled back, quite pleased with myself, even if I didn't want to be mistaken for a lawyer. Sometimes you just have to take those little victories where you can find them.

We brought our baby to the court hearing. She was our

best defense against the world. Balance a baby on your knee and no one will harm you. Bring your baby to the doctor's office, and place a loving husband beside you, and cancer—it wouldn't dare enter the room. A sweet little baby needs its mother. Fate can't be so cruel as to deny her that.

It can be, though.

As the bankrupts before us told their stories to the judge, the room buzzed with the rude chatter of extraneous conversations. Whispered stories of credit card overload, drinking, gambling, bad investments, failed marriages.

As I told our story, a hush fell slowly over the courtroom. One by one, those in the gallery turned their eyes and ears our way. Drama was unfolding—better than television. The judge paused twice to fetch a handkerchief from under her bench. I knew then that our lives were not normal.

An irritating, nagging sensation had been haunting me. "Is this how life is supposed to be?" I asked myself over and over.

"No," the answer rang out firmly, like the bang of a gavel. I was sure of that when we made the judge cry.

She stared down from her bench, wrapped in her black robe, still dabbing at a moist eye with a tissue. She scanned the audience, examining the familiar faces of her regular creditors. On one of them, a muscle twitched, a mouth began to move— he wanted to speak, but she raised an eyebrow and he fell silent. She looked about at the other men in gray business suits and silently dared them to object, but no one did. "Petition granted."

The gavel fell quietly.

"If you sign this paper, you can have your credit card back." He followed us from the courtroom and caught up to us in the hallway. The man from Sears.

"We don't care about our credit card," I chided.

"It won't cost you anything." He held the paper out, confident that it was an offer no one could refuse.

"We don't want our credit card back," I repeated firmly.

We'd like our lives back. Can you give us that, man from Sears?

"Low interest."

The door to the elevator opened and we stepped inside. The man from Sears stayed behind and watched us a moment, hoping we would change our minds.

No? How could they not? he said to himself. How could they pass up such an offer?

He didn't understand.

I watched him scan his list as the elevator door closed, searching for the name of the next debtor to go before the judge.

The repo man came at night to take the Daytona. He didn't have to come then—we wouldn't have given him trouble—but he said he worked best under cover of darkness.

"It's out back," I directed him as I switched on the outside light. "But you don't want it."

"No, I don't," he said, following me down the shadowy walkway. "The bank does."

"They don't really want it, either. They just want to punish us." I handed him the keys. "It has 160,000 miles on it and was hit by a speeding van."

"You're right. They don't want it," he replied. "But I have to take it."

"You want me to turn the porch light on, too?"

He shook his head no. "You're nice people. Most folks get angry."

"We did get angry," I replied. "But not about a car."

He nodded as if he understood. "I have to carry a gun."

"That's too bad," I said as I eyed a suspicious bulge in his shirt. "I don't."

"No, I don't need it with you." He looked at me and I saw he had a tear in his eye. "I don't want to take it, you know." A big burly man whose work alternated between repossessing cars and bouncing drunks at a strip bar, but he had a tear.

"I know," I replied softly.

My wife brought him coffee and I helped hook the Daytona up to his hitch. His mother had died of cancer, he told me after my wife went back into the rented house. Some people tell you about people dying right in front of a sick person, but he didn't.

"It's not the same thing, though," he said. "She was old."

"It's still the same thing," I responded sadly.

"*I*'M COLD." She got up from the sofa by the window. Her sofa, where she would sit each evening and watch the world drive by. She walked down the pink carpeted hallway that led to our pink-walled bedroom.

The house was silent as she searched with her delicate feminine touch through the contents of our shared closet. The door to the bedroom closet closed—loudly, not quietly as it had opened—and she returned.

I had built a small fire in the fireplace. We kept the stone hearth lined with pillows when the fireplace wasn't in use as protection for our young daughter's fragile head. I removed the pillows when I built the fire, because my wife fretted that they would catch fire.

She returned to the living room carrying a sweater, and walked to the fireplace. She looked at the sweater—it was her red-and-white checkered one—and looked into the fire, then casually tossed the sweater into the flames.

"When you said you were cold," I remarked, "I thought you were getting a sweater to wear, not burn."

"I was," she replied. "But then I saw this one, and I had to burn it."

"Why?"

"Because you hate that sweater," she explained. "You almost didn't marry me because of it, and I don't want it around to remind you that you shouldn't have married me." She stared into the fire and watched it burn. It was synthetic and melted first, then burned a deep blue flame.

"Don't be silly," I said. "Of course I should have married you."

"But I've ruined your life." She was crying again. "If you saw the sweater, it would remind you of that, and you'd leave me, just like that politician who left his wife when she had cancer."

"But I'm not a politician. I'm your husband." I stood up from the pink carpeting, then walked to her and hugged her from behind, wrapping my arms around her waist and kissing her ear. "I could cut off my leg if it had cancer, but I could never cut you out of my life."

She spun around and held my chin in her hands, then kissed my lips.

"But I had to burn it. Don't you see? I couldn't feel safe with it here. You say you'll stay, but maybe you won't. Maybe you'll see the sweater, and it will remind you of how you almost didn't marry me, and how if you hadn't, you'd have your house, and your car, and your old job."

She would have continued on, but I shook her gently, and whispered, "But then I wouldn't have you, and I wouldn't have our daughter. I'd have nothing."

She was right. I hated that sweater. She had worn it on our second date—that was the first time I had seen the sweater. It was summer then, and we took the ferry to one of the many islands that dot the New England coast. There we rented bicycles. Halfway up the island's only hill, we bought lemonade from an enterprising young girl whose golden hair stood out—a bold advertisement for her product.

We were walking our bikes at that point, but I still needed a second glass of lemonade to quench my thirst. I paused there on the side of the hill, wiping sweat from my brow and looking off in the direction from which we had come, toward the little fishing port, and thought how beautiful everything looked. I looked toward my date and smiled.

Yes. Everything was so beautiful.

We pushed our bikes to the top of the hill, then climbed back onto their odd-shaped seats and peddled onward, barely needing to move our feet as we rolled with gravity. Heading away from the town, the houses became less and less frequent until we reached a part of the island that had no houses at all. There, we stopped along a beach and looked out across the water.

"Would you like to take a walk?" I asked her.

She nodded yes and got down from her bike.

"Be sure to lock them onto something solid," she said as we leaned the bikes against opposite sides of a sign post.

We walked along the dunes, our feet sinking slightly into the soft beach, our sneakers filling with the loose yellow sand. The beach faced the mainland, not the open ocean, but a stiff breeze blew nonetheless. It was high tide, and the pungent smell of the sea had been dulled by the onslaught of the rising tide.

The land dwindled into a point, grass-covered and solid, except for the cliffs of clay that had collapsed into the pounding surf. On the point of land sat an abandoned lighthouse with a sign nailed to the front door, a sign that asked for volunteers to assemble there the following weekend and work together to save the abandoned lighthouse from the ravages of time.

We stood back from the lighthouse—on the sand beside the lapping waves—and looked up at the vacant hole where a beacon once shone. I moved closer to her and touched her waist with my fingertips. Just a gentle touch. She folded her arms under her chest and kept looking up at the emptiness where the beacon should have been.

Monday came and I returned to work.

"How was the date?" a friend asked.

There had been an ongoing discussion among my colleagues about dating and body language. It was a discussion that had gone on for weeks, dying down at times, almost forgotten at several points until an event—a date, perhaps, or an odd gesture—stimulated interest, and the subject took on a new vigor. My date was a stimulant, and my coworkers gathered near the copy machine to analyze the success of that date.

"Did you . . . do it?" my friend asked eagerly.

"No," I said.

"Did you kiss?" another asked.

"No," I replied more sharply.

"Did you at least hold hands?" a third asked.

"I touched her, but she didn't touch me."

"That's bad," my friend said. "What did she do?"

"She folded her arms," I replied, turning away.

"That's real bad," he said. The others agreed. Bad body language. "Folding her arms—that's rejection. That meant she didn't like you."

I didn't say anything. I stood quietly by, listening to the click of the copy machine, and fought the pain.

She didn't like me.

"She's too old, anyway," my friend remarked flippantly. "She can't have children. Forget about her."

I tried to forget about her. I didn't talk to her for three weeks, but I couldn't forget her. I knew we belonged together. Finally, I called her on the telephone. "Would you like to go out this weekend?"

"Yes," she said. That was all. Yes.

The weekend came, and I went to her apartment to pick her up. There was no doorbell, so I tapped gently on her door.

The outside light went on.

She opened her apartment door and threw her arms around me. She kissed me with a passion that told me yes, yes, yes. She knew, too. We belonged together.

We were older than most when we married, and we were patient. We had waited for true love. I wasted my youth searching bars and drinking too much until one day I stared in horror at the dark tunnel that lay ahead that was my future, and looked behind and saw the dim receding light that was my past. I groped and crawled, scratching out of the dark depths to which I'd fallen, and entered once again into the light—and there she was, patiently waiting for me.

What took you so long? She spoke without words, for we shared the same soul.

I was lost, but now I've found you, I silently replied.

We married quickly and decided to have a family quickly, but nature was not so kind.

"I'm so sorry," she cried. "I'm just too old to have a baby." She sat on the edge of our bed, examining the stick from a home pregnancy test. "I waited too long."

"You waited for me," I replied softly.

"I had to," she said. "You weren't there before."

"Don't worry. I'll get you pregnant."

"No. You can't." She shook her head. Too old. Too old. Too old.

"Come." I took her hand. "Let's keep trying."

She smiled broadly. "That's all you men think about."

We were patient. She was anxious, I was optimistic, but together we were patient. And tucked somewhere in her body lay a patient egg waiting optimistically for an anxious sperm, and we had our patient baby. A baby that waited too patiently until even the doctor couldn't stand it any longer, and he went in after her with a scalpel to fetch her out through my wife's belly button.

After the baby was born, she was going through her old clothes, looking for something that would fit. She held up the red-and-white checkered sweater.

"Not that one," I said.

"Why not?" she asked.

I told her about the ferry ride and the bike ride and how she folded her arms. I told her about body language.

"See?" I said. "That's why I didn't call you."

"My feelings were hurt when you didn't call."

"I thought you didn't like me," I replied. "You folded your arms."

"I was cold," she explained. "That was all. I was cold."

Now she was cold again, and left the living room of the rented house to find a sweater to wear. But once more, she had found the red-and-white checkered one, folded and forgotten in the back of a closet, not seen since the pregnancy, and she brought it to the living room and tossed it into the fire.

"You shouldn't have burned it," I said as I watched it melt and drip slowly over the log.

"But we both hated it," she cried.

"It was like an heirloom, though," I explained. I pointed to the little girl playing on the pink carpet. "When she got older, we could have given it to her and told her the story, and it would have gotten passed down to future generations, along with the family pants."

"But we hated it," she sighed.

It was our Fort Ticonderoga. A bit of history, but its history was too recent. It was painful for us—not a place to be revisited. Not yet, anyway. But it had been carted away before we had a chance to realize that it was a part of who we were. It was gone before we had a chance to preserve it for the future.

Chapter 5

❧

"See. It's coming in curly." She stood before the bathroom mirror and ran her fingers through her hair.

"It is curly," I agreed. I threaded my fingers through her short hair until our two palms met and our fingers intertwined. "There's no gray, either."

"That will come later." She laughed. "This is my $20,000 perm." She rubbed the short wet hair with a towel and kept rubbing, happy to feel something between the towel and her scalp again. "Of course, I'll still wear a wig in public so people won't stare."

"They'll think you're exotic, with your hair so short," I said. "Someone dark and artistic."

"No, they'll stare."

"They'll think you're a poet."

"Poetess," she replied.

"Poet," I said, smiling at my own little joke.

"You!" she shouted playfully, and rubbed my long hair with her damp towel.

Earlier, when her hair first fell out, I thought of having my head shaved. Camaraderie. But time slipped by, and I never had it cut, let alone shaved.

"Do you think it will fall out again with the radiation?" she asked anxiously as she examined the little curls more closely in the steam-shrouded mirror.

"No, they'll radiate the breast, not your head."

"But those movies, the ones where there's a nuclear war. The people get sick and their hair falls out."

"That's different," I replied.

"Then they die," she said. "That's not different."

"You're not going to die," I assured her. "You'll live to be a hundred."

She stopped rubbing her damp hair, peeked out from under the white towel, and looked off into an uncertain future that only she could fathom. "What will happen to me?" she asked. "And to the two of you afterward?"

I looked into the hallway at our daughter playing on the pink carpeting. "If we're all good, we'll get Christmas presents. That's what will happen."

The little girl seemed to understand. She giggled, and a bubble formed on her upper lip, then burst.

"But we have no money," my wife complained. "We can have a tree this year, though, can't we? And ornaments?"

"You'll be our Christmas ornament this year," I laughed. "They'll radiate your breast and you'll glow like Rudolph, only it won't be your nose."

Her face darkened, and she was about to cry.

"I'm sorry," I replied. "That wasn't funny. You've had your privacy invaded enough without me hanging you out as an ornament."

"It's not that," she murmured sadly. "It's just I've ruined your life, you know."

"Nonsense, love," I responded. "You are my life."

"But you've lost your house and your dog, and now you won't have a Christmas, and it's all because I got sick."

"But getting sick wasn't your fault," I explained. "And we lost the house because of the lousy economy. You had nothing to do with that."

She smiled as she took my hand, but she said no more.

We walked from the bathroom and followed our daughter as she crawled quickly forward, leading the way to the living room and the spot where we would put our Christmas tree.

"Just some little presents so the tree won't look so sad," she said—asked—as she looked at the bare window where the tree would go. "There doesn't have to be anything in them. Just some pretty boxes. Except for her." She nodded toward our daughter. "We can get something for her, can't we?"

I reached into my back pocket and pulled out my wallet. "Here," I said as I whipped out a JC Penny charge card. "I've been saving this one for an emergency."

"But the bankruptcy?" she asked, startled.

"There was no balance on this one," I explained. "So the account stayed open."

That evening, we sat side-by-side on the living room sofa, wedged together against its padded arm. A borrowed copy of the JC Penny Christmas catalog sat sprawled across our unified laps. I smiled at my wife as I watched her fingers flip through the pages of the catalog. They never stopped on a women's page, never paused to let her admire a blouse or catch the alluring scent of perfume, but instead searched for gifts for others.

"Which one do you like?" she asked as we stared down at a page full of men outfitted in snowflake sweaters.

I smiled. "I don't need a sweater. You keep me warm."

Her fingers darted forward, to the toy section. "Can we get her more than one thing?" she asked cheerfully.

"Get her whatever you like."

"Of course, there's more to Christmas than presents," she observed.

"That's true," I replied.

"But she's just a little girl and it would be a shame if we didn't make her first real Christmas something special."

Christmas wasn't white that year. It was festive enough, though. Reds. Greens. My wife wore a green-and-red bandanna even though Christmas was with family and they wouldn't have stared at her short hair.

Blues, yellows, and oranges, too. I decorated our tree with strings of tiny lights, the inexpensive ones where the entire string goes dark when one bulb burns out. Each evening, I would find another darkened string, and I would sit before the fireplace, leaning against the protective pillows, testing light bulbs until I found the culprit and restored the string to a festive glow.

"Why is that string blinking?" she asked casually as she sat on her sofa, browsing through her holiday cookbook.

"I was out of regular bulbs," I explained. "So I put in one of those blinker lights."

"It would be okay if just one light blinked, but it looks like a bar when the whole string blinks on and off together."

I took the offending bulb out and the entire string went dark.

"That's better," she said.

"I'll get the right kind tomorrow," I assured her with a smile. She was concerned about blinking lights, worried about appetizers and hungry guests, and, oh yes. . .

"Did you water the tree?" she suddenly asked.

"No," I said.

"You don't want it to dry out."

She was worried about dried trees. Christmas was a holiday of hope more than anything else. Perhaps, for a few days, she could feel that hope, understand normal pleasures again, and not be burdened by what always lurked in the background, like a cobweb dangling in the corner of the room—a spider, and we were its prey.

Christmas day—after the guests left—we kissed under the mistletoe, while our daughter played noisily in the large pile of discarded wrapping paper.

"It was a wonderful Christmas," my wife uttered. "Thank you."

"I'm glad you liked it."

Tears welled up in her eyes, and she started to cry.

"What's wrong, honey?" I asked.

"Nothing," she replied. "I just love you for making my last Christmas so wonderful."

"No, not your last," I whispered softly in her ear as I held her tight against me. "You're going to live to be a hundred."

We watched quietly as our daughter stuck bows to her hair and, giggling, draped ribbons over her shoulders. We both saw the irony, the child playing in the gift wrap, and the presents— the presents that we could barely afford—sitting ignored beside the tree.

"Next year we'll just wrap empty boxes for her to play with," my wife said as she strolled to the glass punchbowl and scooped a cup of the now-diluted eggnog out from beside a huge floating ice cube.

Next year. She was talking about next year. I had gotten my Christmas wish after all.

Chapter 6

❧

*I*T BARELY SNOWED the winter of 1992. That was good, since the Daytona was gone and the Firebird was old. The Judge let us keep the Firebird because it was paid for and had little value. She let us keep it because we had made her cry. The brakes didn't work very well, though, so my brother-in-law and I struggled to fix them.

"Should they be leaking fluid like that?" I asked as I stared at his feet sticking out from beside the rear tire.

"They'll be fine," he replied, his feet jerking as he grappled with an unseen nut. "Just be sure to check the reservoir occasionally."

The brakes never were quite right after that, so we used the car sparingly. Each morning, I walked to the train station. Down the short cut, along the railroad tracks. It was a cold winter, but only once did it snow hard. The snow from that one storm, though, remained stubbornly on the ground through all of January and halfway into February.

With the freight trains, I barely noticed the lack of snowfall. Passing box cars created their own brew of winter havoc— fast moving high pressure systems in their own right.

A locomotive snuck up silently, the sound of its massive engine muffled by the vast expanse of snow, the blast of its horn arriving almost too late to warn me. I jumped off the track to the safety of the access road, and stood watching—amazed— as it passed. It rattled me about, almost spinning me around like a top as it engulfed me in a blizzard of its own making. Then it was gone, and there was silence. In the distance, I heard a thud as a squirrel knocked a pine cone from the top of an evergreen. Snow could be funny, with the big things so silent, while the little things . . . thud.

Even after the snow had grown old and crusted over, the power of the freight trains tore at it, ripped it from the ground, pulverized it, and whipped it about my face.

I thought of my grandfather. "When I was a boy, I had to walk nine miles to school, through three-foot drifts. . ." How true was that? It's hard to say. Time alters the past. I remember walking to the train station day after day through fields of snow, but I also remember that it only snowed once.

On days when the wind blew cold, I dreamed idly of building myself a mail hook—like they showed on those old westerns. I could hang myself outside our bedroom window each morning, bobbing up and down in my elastic suspenders until the passing commuter train plucked me off and hauled me safely into Boston.

Coming home, in the winter darkness, there were eyes all about, watching me. Walking the tracks, sometimes tip-toeing along, balancing on the steel rails like a school kid, at other times struggling on the ties that were spaced wrong for my long stride, I could see the eyes staring out at me from the ice-choked wetlands.

Bobcats? Mountain lions? Bears! I visualized the headline. "Man mauled to death along train tracks." Or were they eyes of . . . that? Evil eyes from unearthly creatures, the disciples of disease, spreading fear, keeping an watch on me—sentries— while their fellow tormentors were back at the rented house gnawing at my wife, at her breast, at her life.

I quickened my pace, but then I saw that they were the small frightened eyes of woodland creatures, many that would not survive the harsh winter.

"You should get boots," she said as I entered the house. "Your feet must be cold."

"I walk on the tracks, not in the snow," I replied, stamping the snow from my shoes.

"What about trains?" She brushed the snow from my parka, and pointed to our daughter. She wanted to say, "You might get hit by a train." But the words were too powerful, the image was too real, too frightening. Things like that did happen. She couldn't say it, and instead whispered, "She'd be an orphan."

"It's a single track," I explained. "Nothing can come back down the track until the commuter train clears Lawrence."

"I just worry so much about you," she sighed. "You don't want our daughter to be an orphan."

Once, I saw the form of a man walking toward me in the darkness. That frightened me more than the animal eyes, more than rogue trains. A man! Out there on those desolate train tracks, shadowy against the snow and indistinct under the hazy moonlight, out where there was no one to witness our meeting. We passed each other with downcast eyes, each thinking the same thing, each knowing that the other was thinking the same thing—"What is he doing out here?"

Most nights, though, it was the eyes of hungry little crea-tures that stared out at me. I was going home, to a warm house and a loving wife, to my sweet young daughter. I was lucky. The animals were cold, and I was lucky.

"We were lucky it didn't snow this winter," I remarked as I placed my winter coat in a box.

"We'll pay for it next year," she replied, carefully folding a sweater.

We were packing our belongings. Moving. The owner of the raised ranch wanted to sell it. My wife was doing chemother-apy again. 5-FU pumped slowly and steadily into her veins from a little fanny pack. Every fifteen minutes, the hushed whirl of the little machine told us medicine was coming. Poison.

She didn't feel good. Mouth sores, fatigue. And the real estate agents kept calling with the same question. "What time would be convenient to show the house?"

Convenient? Summertime would be convenient. Autumn would be even better.

We had a reliable car again, so we no longer needed to live near the train station. A minivan. We had been saving money. Ramen Pride noodles for lunch for six months. They cost six-teen cents a serving and came in four flavors. I was a vegetar-ian, so I stuck to mushroom flavor. We saved, and with my Christmas bonus, we had enough to start thinking about get-ting a car.

"We can spend $4500," I told the car salesman as I exam-ined a late model sedan.

"This one's a beauty," the salesman replied. "Only $6500."

"We can only spend $4500," I reminded him as a stepped over to the next vehicle.

He waved off my remark. "This one here is in your price range. Only $7200. Asking price. You can finance."

"My wife has cancer," I explained. "We just went through bankruptcy, and we only have $4500."

His salesman's smile faded, and he took us to the back of the lot, behind the auto body shop. "This one just came in. I was saving it for myself. I'll talk to the boss and see what we can do."

"A minivan," my wife commented as she peered into the roomy interior. "I wasn't thinking of a van. I was thinking we'd get a sedan."

"Is it okay, though?" I asked anxiously.

She stood back from it and scanned its exterior with a critical eye. A van.

No, not a van—a minivan.

"Do you have to shift it or anything?" she asked suspiciously.

"No. It's just like driving a car." I smiled. "Except a bell rings when you back up."

She laughed.

"There's no air conditioning," she said as we sat together in the front seat and examined the dashboard.

"We'll drive into the mountains when it gets hot," I suggested.

"It will hold a lot of stuff," she observed.

That was important with an infant. Diaper bags. Cribs. High chairs. Play pens. There was no traveling light when you had an infant.

"If I feel better this summer, and it gets hot, we could go camping in the mountains. Couldn't we?" she pleaded.

Her doctor did his part to make her feel better.

"Your breast is nice and supple again," he commented. "It's really miraculous."

He disconnected the tube that led from the fanny pack to

the place in her chest where they had implanted the porta-cathal shunt—a little drum device for taking blood out and pouring medical stuff in—toxins, mostly.

"It's important that you eat," he explained. He had examined her mouth sores and her breast. He weighed the two in his medical mind. She was supple again, but she couldn't eat, so it was time to stop the treatment.

"But what about the liver?" she asked anxiously.

"The liver's fine," her doctor replied.

"But the other doctor. . ."

Ignore the other doctor. He was a jerk. That's why we're in Boston.

Her Boston doctor held up two X-rays. Liver scans. Before and after. No change. It was a hemangioma all along. Not a tumor. "You've probably had it since birth," he surmised.

"See, honey," I assured her. "You'll live to be a hundred."

We returned to our packing with a new sense of optimism.

"Do you think he's right about the liver?" she asked as she began filling a second box with sweaters.

"Of course he's right about the liver," I answered, taping the lid shut on our daughter's toys.

"Because if he is right, maybe there's a chance I'll be. . ." But her voice trailed off. She wanted to say it, but she couldn't even dare to think it.

Cured.

Chapter 7

≈

W E MOVED from the rented house by the railroad tracks to an apartment complex. Luxury apartments, with a swimming pool, an exercise room, air conditioning, saunas, and a hot tub.

It was the day before our wedding anniversary, one year since the diagnosis of her illness. I held a bouquet behind my back and slid quietly through the front door.

"She's turning into a little person," my wife remarked cheerfully. She knew I was there, but she didn't turn to greet me. Instead, she watched our daughter as she played on the floor. "She was so sweet as a baby," my wife continued. "But now that she's almost two, you can see her becoming a little person, and I like that even more."

"That's because the baby is nature's work, but the little person is your doing," I replied as I walked toward her. "You can see all your efforts rewarded in her."

My wife had worked twenty years for an insurance company, but she left after we were married. At first, she seemed embarrassed to be a homemaker. When we met other couples, and the wives introduced themselves as the assistant to the CEO or the deputy commissioner for employee relations, she introduced herself by her former title.

Once our daughter was born, that changed. It was okay to stay at home then. Rock, paper, scissors. Career girl, wife, motherhood.

It was more than okay. It was a noble cause. Civilizing a little being, as my wife called it, implanting her years of learning into a young mind—a mind that was like a sponge and soaked up everything.

The little girl spotted the bouquet of flowers before my wife did, and pointed to them, shouting "boo-bay."

"You shouldn't have," my wife remarked, a slight smile contradicting her words as she looked up and saw the flowers. "We're trying to save our money."

"I could try growing you flowers in a litter box or something," I said with a laugh. "But it's spring, and flowers are cheap in Boston."

She took the bouquet and handed me a drawing in exchange. Our daughter had drawn it with her crayons. "This is what she wants on her birthday cake."

"A yellow tonsil?"

"It's Big Bird." She laughed as she took a tall vase from the dining room buffet and laid the flowers out on the dining room table. "From Sesame Street. See the orange? That's its beak."

I watched in awe as she converted the pile of assorted flowers into a work of art. She never put flowers in a random vase.

She would eye the bouquet, size it up for color and character, then carefully select the proper vase from her vast collection. She didn't jam the entire bouquet into the vase, but took up each stalk individually, examined it, clipped it to the proper length, and placed it in the vase perfectly.

"You've got such a talent," I observed. "You should design flower arrangements from home."

"You want me to go back to work?"

"No," I said. "I just want you to do something you enjoy."

She smiled and look over at our daughter tossing crayons into the air.

No, she was complete. Her flower arrangements would be for her and for me. She had no desire to prove her talent to the outside world. No need anymore of insurance companies. No need for itchy wool suits and Gucci briefcases. Motherhood had made her everything she wanted to be.

I stared at the picture that my wife had handed to me. "Oh, I see it now. There's the beak, and there's the feet."

"I think that's the eye." She took up a sprig of baby's breath and placed it so that the delicate white flowers hung down over the rim of the pressed glass vase. "She's quite a little artist, don't you think?"

"She's wonderful," I said as I smiled at our daughter. "She takes after you."

"Bib bood." The little girl laughed as she worked at her new creation with a blue crayon, something akin to a dehydrated plum.

"Grover?" I asked, recalling another Sesame Street character. Now that I knew the theme, I had a fighting chance at interpreting my daughter's artwork.

The little girl smiled and nodded yes.

"The cake shouldn't be too hard to make," my wife explained as she slipped a daffodil into the center of the vase. "Big Bird is mostly yellow."

She had taken a cake decorating class during the tail end of her treatment, something that was not too strenuous, but would restore to her a sense of being part of life. She learned how to decorate cakes, but more importantly, she learned she didn't like to decorate cakes. She passed her new skills on to me, and I was now the family cake decorator.

"I'll need a better picture of bib bood." I looked toward our daughter to see if she had heard me, had noticed my gentle teasing. She hadn't. She was too busy. Her head was bobbing back and forth as a purple dinosaur sang and danced his way across the television screen.

"There." My wife placed a blue iris so that its white mantle faced outward. She centered the vase on the dining room table, then brought me a paper bag. "Use this." She had purchased a cake mold shaped like Big Bird. Pasted on the inside were the decorating instructions. "I wanted you to see her picture first. It's so cute."

After dinner, I put the Big Bird cake mold away—our daughter's birthday was not for three months. Living with cancer was like living in a department store—we grabbed onto an event to occupy our minds, and started celebrating far ahead in case she didn't make it. It was late spring, but we were already planning late summer birthdays. The following month, we would be sewing Halloween costumes. And we would be out tagging a Christmas tree while others were picking out their pumpkins.

"You'll remember where you put it?" my wife asked as she watched me stash Big Bird behind my abandoned garden tools.

"You'll remind me," I said.

"If I'm still here," she replied solemnly.

"You'll live to be a hundred," I replied, smiling, as I fetched our gym bag, ready to embark on our evening workout.

My wife was feeling stronger. No more chemotherapy, no more radiation. Just a daily dose of tamoxifen—some sort of hormone treatment that couldn't be fully explained.

"Sometimes it works," her doctor explained. "We don't really know why."

"Do you think it will help me?" she asked.

"You tumor marker is dropping," he replied excitedly, referring to the blood test he did each month to count tumor-produced proteins. If that count went down, it meant the tumors were shrinking. In theory.

Everything was in theory.

"If I build up my strength, I should be able to fight off the cancer better," my wife suggested.

Yes. In theory.

So we started to exercise.

The apartment complex had a small health club with rowing machines, stationery bicycles, Stairmasters.

We left the apartment after dinner, holding hands, the three of us—mother, father, and daughter.

Outside, a man's buttocks stared out the window of the downstairs apartment, his feet kicking about in the air. My wife and I looked at each other, but we said nothing until we had walked out of sight. Then we shook our heads and laughed.

Chapter 8

🖎

*T*HE SUMMER HEAT CAME. My wife stayed inside, in the air-conditioned comfort of the apartment. I returned home from work to find my daughter standing nearby, in the shadows, waiting for me.

"Play with me, Dada?"

Yes, my pumpkin.

"She's too young to swim," my wife remarked anxiously. "She's not even two."

We stood by the front doorway in our bathing suits—beach towels draped over our shoulders—ready to walk the short distance to the swimming pool.

"You've got to start them early." I puffed some air into the limp plastic tubes that encased my daughter's upper arms, and the tubes plumped out in response. "Besides, she's got her water wings on."

"Just be careful," my wife warned. "Keep an eye on her."

Keep an eye on her? I intended to keep a hand on her, never let her slip from my grasp. Hold her, protect her, love her.

"Sure you don't want to come, too?" I asked.

She shook her head. Too hot. Her thermostat had broken— it had suffered some sort of a meltdown in the course of radiation treatments. She was always either too hot or too cold.

The little girl was impatient and wouldn't pause long enough for me to slip her into her sandals. Outside, even with the sun approaching the horizon, the sidewalk was hot against her tender feet, and she had to walk in the cool grass. The parking areas were lined with decorative rocks, and she climbed over each one as I held her hand. Her hand was locked in mine—a little flower—as we entered the gated pool area.

"It's adult swim," the lifeguard called over as we set our towels in a plastic chair. "She can't go in."

"Adult swim?" I asked.

"Yes. Six until closing on weeknights is adult swim." She twirled her whistle, a symbol of her authority. "Eighteen and over only."

"I work all day." I hopped into the pool, sweeping my daughter from the deck of the pool and into my arms. "I can't get here before six."

I felt a brief moment of regret. She was obviously a teenager—the pimple cream cracked around the corners of her lips as her blank expression turned into a frown. She must have defied her parents for years, but was now emerging from that defiance and learning responsibility. Now I came along and defied her—a bad example. Oh well, she'll heal.

She went for reinforcements—maleness to overcome her

femaleness. But it wasn't that which made me disobey—it wasn't that she was a girl. It was that the rule was wrong.

The apartment manager marched from the rear door of the clubhouse, slapping across the wet patio in his Chinese sandals. "It's adult swim." He stood hovering over me as I floated beneath him in the cool water, his feet straddling where "no diving" was painted on the edge of the pool deck. "She has to be eighteen."

The lifeguard waited quietly beside him, feeling her confidence return as she stood in the shadow of this handsome young man.

"I work all day," I explained. "Evenings are the only time we can swim together."

Apparently some adults didn't like children, and the apartment manager wished to cater to that group. But there was no modest bathing suit swim for those who disapproved of jiggling flesh and skimpy strips of cloth stuck between cracks and cleavage. No sixty and under swim for those who didn't wish to be reminded of the degenerative power of time. The only people management wished to cater to were those who disliked swimming among children.

"She can swim during the day," he suggested, struggling to suppress the urge to tap an impatient foot at me.

"No she can't," I replied. "I work."

Adult swim. The entire evening. Half an hour, even an hour—I could have worked around that. But the entire evening reserved for those with an odd aversion to children? I couldn't let that stand.

"A father with an eighteen-year-old son," I asked. "Could he go swimming with his son right now?"

"Yes," the manager replied, tossing his young blond hair about with confidence.

"But I have a two-year-old daughter, so I can't." I swung

my daughter up over my head, bringing her eye-to-eye with the manager so he could see her sweet innocent face.

"That's right." He began to see the path we were taking. He stopped tossing his head about as his confidence waned.

"And does the father with the eighteen-year-old pay more rent than I do?"

My daughter giggled in response as though she also knew where I was headed. But out of the corner of my eye, I saw the umbrella spinning slowly in the breeze above the poolside table and knew that was what amused her.

"Of course not." He stood still. He slid his hands into his pockets as he waited patiently for the knockout punch.

"Then why are they entitled to more services than I am?"

Victory.

He turned and whispered a few words to the lifeguard, then returned to the clubhouse doors, his sandals slapping harder against the concrete than they had on the way out. The lifeguard watched the young man go, disappointed. She would not sleep with him now. She glanced at me, then strolled to her chair and began spinning her whistle, the universal lifeguard sign that all was well. Nobody said anything to me directly. They surrendered in silence.

I placed my daughter on my stomach and slowly kicked to the middle of the pool, blowing a spout of water from my mouth like a whale. I felt refreshed.

Two children appeared by the gate, a brother and a sister. They locked their bikes and grabbed their beach towels from the handlebars.

The lifeguard snatched her spinning whistle from the air and popped it in her mouth, ready for action. But she did not blow. "Adult swim," she called, pulling the whistle from her mouth, but holding it near her lips in case a quick toot was needed to repel the small invaders. "Eighteen and over."

"Why can she swim then?" They pointed at my daughter.

"Because she's with her father," the lifeguard replied.

"If we get our father. . ."

No. You had to be under two. That was their new rule, she explained. Less than two years old and adults only.

Jesus Christ, let the kids swim, I wanted to yell. But I had made enough trouble for one day, and remained silent, hoping that common sense would prevail. After all, there was no one in the pool other than me and my daughter. Adults didn't want a swim after a hard day at work. They wanted a beer. They wanted the news, a good meal, a better lay, and a final burp.

Common sense did not win out that day, though. The two children watched me from beside their bicycles, grinding their toes into the ground. Envy, hope—I don't know what their child minds were thinking—but they soon grew bored. I barely heard them as they climbed onto their bikes and pedaled away.

Afterward, we strolled homeward, refreshed from our hard-won swim. I held my sneakers in one hand and my daughter's hand in the other as we walked barefoot in the cool shadows of the parking lot.

She climbed a rock. "I love you, Dada." She stretched up on her toes but was still too small to reach my cheek.

"I love you, too," I replied, lifting her from the rock and to my chest.

Her smile broadened. "I love you more."

"I love you the most."

"I love you like toast."

"I love you from coast to coast."

I set her down. Together, we ran across the damp evening grass toward the front door of the apartment building. She reached up with her small fingers, but could not reach the buzzer to our apartment.

I gave her a little boost.

"Who is it?" My wife's voice crackled from the small speaker.

"It is us," I replied. "Your water bugs have returned."

Luxury living. The neighbors downstairs gave new meaning to the term "dysfunctional."

"We can't sleep at night," I complained to the apartment manager. "They stay up all night screaming obscenities back and forth."

"They used to do it in the parking lot," he replied, once again tossing his blond hair confidently about, our recent poolside meeting already a distant memory. "Thankfully, we got them to move it indoors."

"That doesn't help if you live over them."

It went on for months, then one day the boyfriend was gone.

"We got rid of the boyfriend for you," the manager said with a smile.

I was supposed to smile back, but I didn't. "She's got new boyfriends now," I replied.

"Boyfriends?" he asked. "How many?"

"Too many to count." I sat opposite his desk and waited for a reaction, but he said nothing. "They come after midnight and pound on her bedroom window."

"They pound on her window?"

"Yes. Then she opens it and they crawl in," I explained. "And when they're through, they crawl back out."

He jotted a note on a scrap of paper. "We can speak to her again."

"Then they'll bang on the ceiling," I replied.

"She bangs her boyfriends on the ceiling?" He was trying to be funny, but I didn't laugh.

"No, they bang in her bed," I said. "She bangs on the ceiling with a broom handle if we complain."

"We can't get rid of her." He twirled his pencil but wrote no further. "The welfare agency will say you're prejudiced."

Our neighbor was French Canadian. My wife's maiden name was French Canadian. They could have been long-lost cousins—but the agency would say we were prejudiced.

"Prejudiced against people who have boyfriends climbing through their window and who bang on their ceilings?"

"No," he explained. "Against people on welfare."

Luxury apartments. The developer used government money to build the place, and in return the government made them take in welfare people at reduced rates. Into luxury apartments.

We had ignored the advice of friends who had told us not to move there, that it was full of welfare recipients. But we had known poverty, and had been victimized by those random uncontrollable events that can cast you into financial ruin. Good people do fail.

"He said they're doing all they can to get her out." I picked our daughter up from the floor and saw the meticulous cleanliness of the carpeting. Grinning, I looked at my wife. "You vacuumed again."

"They kept me up all night again," she complained. "You never hear it."

"I heard it, but I fell back asleep."

"I couldn't fall back asleep," she replied. "So I vacuumed."

It was justice. If my wife couldn't sleep, our neighbor shouldn't sleep. The bedroom was always cleanest. That was where she vacuumed first, knowing that the woman lay directly below, sprawled across her deranged bed, rattling her scarred arms among a collection of crumpled beer cans and used condoms, hung over and naked.

I would kiss my wife good-bye, and then she would start up the vacuum. I'd hear it roar to life as I walked down the stairs, and I would smile. She was fretting—fretting about noisy neighbors; fretting about immoral sex and illegal drugs; fretting about things the rest of us fret about. Free, for a moment, at least, from the worry that was always there, lurking somewhere in the background. Haunting us.

She developed new skills—human radar. She no longer needed to turn the vacuum off to hear where the woman was hiding. The soles of her feet could sense the rattle of the woman's coffee cup as she struggled against a hangover in the dining room below. Right . . . about . . . there . . . and my wife would vacuum our dining room—directly overhead.

The woman would move to the living room, sit quietly in the corner chair, curl her legs up into her chest and hug her shivering body. But the squeak of the cushion, the exhaling of cigarette smoke—it would give her away, and my wife would move the vacuum into our living room, run the noisy power nozzle back and forth across the woman's throbbing forehead.

But then a sound—the woman puking in the bathroom—and my wife would stop. She knew the feeling. She could sympathize with it, even if the cause was not the same. Even if the woman below did not deserve sympathy, illness did.

You've won the battle, my love. Lay down your arms.

The vacuum fell silent.

Chapter 9

᯽

SHE NEEDED REST, but wasn't getting it at home. We retreated into the wilderness, stuffing the van with a tent and sleeping bags, a Coleman stove and fishing poles, r a rubber raft, goggles, snorkels. Sand chairs, saltines, and a battery-powered radio. Band-Aids, mercurochrome, and a tourniquet. No snake bite kit.

We camped in Maine along the Moose River, outside of Jackman, a town which was little more than a lumber camp with a Laundromat and a post office.

"This must be a tributary," I commented as we stood on the edge of our campsite and watched the trickle of water run past our feet.

It wasn't a tributary, though. There had been a drought, and the Moose River was dry. The drought broke that night. Other campers around us abandoned ship as the river began to rise, swallowing up the low-lying campsites, filling them with the thick brown saliva of a hungry river.

The three of us huddled in the dampness of our little tent until the morning sun broke through and rewarded us for our patience.

I took our daughter for a ride in the rubber raft. She said she wanted to go, but when she saw the image of her mother standing on the riverbank beside the swollen river, and saw that image growing smaller and smaller as the rapid current dragged us further and further away, she began to cry.

I landed the raft at an abandoned dock and carried her through the dripping forest until we emerged from the trees and startled my wife.

"She missed you," I explained.

Silently, she took the child from my arms and kissed her.

We stood quietly and watched the water swirl where no water had been before. She turned her face toward mine and tried to smile.

"I love you," she said.

The weekend ended, and we returned home to chaos. In our absence, the woman below had brawled with another tenant and tensions ran high.

My wife scoured the travel section of the Sunday paper while her coffee cooled beside her, yearning for some peaceful spot. "It's been a long time since we had a real vacation," she remarked.

"Where would you like to go?" I asked cautiously.

"Someplace cool," she replied. "Maine, maybe. We could go camping in Maine again, only this time for a whole week." She thought for a moment about what she had just said. "We won't stay in a tent because a week is too long to stay in a tent."

"In a cabin?" I asked.

"That's what I had in mind." She set the newspaper aside—we were not discussing the luxury getaways that were splashed across the travel section in enticing color.

"Would it still be camping?" I asked.

"If the cabin is rustic enough," she assured me. "And we'll cook outside. That will make it camping."

"We'll have to sleep on the floor, though," I teased. "Even if the cabin has beds. Right?"

We watched the sky. For two weeks we could look through the night air directly up at our small galaxy—the stars, the moon, a meteor streaking across the horizon.

"That's an airplane," she explained.

Oh.

She grabbed a loaf of bread from the back of the van, rescuing it from my careless handling. I lifted out the rest of the groceries, while our daughter carried only her doll Sally.

"Another clear night," my wife said, saddened to see good weather wasted on a work night.

Come daylight, the clear blue sky. A rare cloud, its smallness flitting across the parking lot like the shadow of a bird.

She fretted about the beautiful sky as it unfolded amid the sunrise. "Too many nice days," she'd say, looking out through the living room window. "That's twelve days in a row. It'll have to rain on us."

Then Saturday morning, the first day of vacation—fog. We drove north on the interstate. I slouched in the driver's seat, squinting toward the east, searching for the blue that had so recently dominated the sky, but it was gone. Out to sea. Perhaps to Europe by now, enjoyed by pudgy Russians lounging along the Black Sea in their thong bathing suits as they contemplated capitalism.

Like the Russians, I too shifted my gaze west, looking for a sign that the fine weather would soon return.

But it rained the entire week. Never enough to ruin the day, but just enough so we were always looking up, searching for a break in the clouds.

The campground director looked out at the bored faces of the campers, and frowned seeing them huddled in their tents, trying to keep warm and dry. He cranked up the heat in the swimming pool until steam drifted off the water's surface, luring the campers from their dreary tents and into the water.

"Don't let her get cold," my wife warned as my daughter and I changed into our bathing suits. We too had fallen victim to the allure of the rising steam.

"The water's ninety-five degrees," I argued. "We won't get cold."

"You won't, but she's little. Just watch her. If you see her shiver. . ."

I placed my daughter on my shoulders and set off down the dirt trail at a jog, toward the swimming pool.

We entered the pool quickly—chilled from the jog through the cool, misty rain—and knelt down to let the heat of the water warm us.

I wanted my daughter to stick her face in the water, to take a step closer to being a true swimmer, so I told her there were sea shells on the bottom of the pool.

"Where, Dada?"

"They're white. They're hard to see against the white cement," I explained. "You have to put your face in the water."

Sometimes it's okay for a parent to lie to a child. Little white lies. Harmless parent lies.

She pinched her nose as she dipped her head into the steamy water, then returned quickly to the surface. "Oh yeah. I saw one," she claimed, her eyes still closed from their brief encounter with the water.

I laughed. A child lie for a parent lie.

We cooked inside because of the rain—on a stove discarded

by its original owner, salvaged from a scrap pile and brought to a summer camp, then discarded again and brought to this cabin, leaning oddly on an uneven floor against a backdrop of exposed two-by-fours and knotty pine clapboard. Its enamel was chipped, but otherwise it was in working order.

"I guess that means this isn't a camping trip," I said as I fried our morning eggs in a dark cast-iron skillet.

She slid up behind me and kissed the back of my neck. "Is it so bad being cooped up with me?"

I turned my head and smiled. "No. It's the way a vacation should be."

She moved toward the window and looked out at the grayness that had settled onto everything. "Perhaps the sun will come out tomorrow," she said. "Then you can cook breakfast outside."

She said that again each evening as she cooked dinner—perhaps the sun will come out tomorrow—but it never did. Not until the last evening. Then briefly, the sun did come out—just before sunset—and everybody ran from their campfires to the beach, staring up like an alien spaceship was descending from the heavens.

"We'll just make the best of it," she vowed as we sat facing each other in a rented rowboat, trolling for fish in the middle of the lake.

The early morning fog had turned to late-morning drizzle. We clutched our rain gear tighter around our necks and tossed our fishing lines less frequently into the surrounding water.

We caught nothing.

"I thought the fishing was supposed to be good in the rain," I complained.

"Not with you two sitting in the back of the boat singing, 'It's raining, it's pouring,'" my wife sighed.

We drifted down a small river in our inflatable raft, moisture dripping from the leaves overhead, marking the water with concentric rings, confusing us. Was it still raining or not? Stopping along the riverbank for a picnic, we climbed up into an open field of a small park. No, it was not raining. The highway ran alongside the field, high above on a grassy embankment so that the park still had a feeling of seclusion. At noon, despite the threat of rain, three pickup trucks with oversized tires rattled down a dirt trail. We were joined in the picnic grove by half a dozen road workers in yellow hard hats, eating bologna sandwiches and drinking Budweisers discreetly out of paper bags.

After lunch, we pointing the raft upstream, but found the current too hard to paddle against. I hopped into the water and pulled the raft back up the river by its rope, my wife and daughter sitting uncomfortably on the raft's wet bottom. I hung the rope over my shoulder and imagined I was Humphrey Bogart and the raft was the African Queen.

Vacation ended. I sighed in relief—we had run out of rainy day adventures long before we had run out of rainy days. I packed our luggage into the back of the van. The rain stopped, and the sun broke out in a way that let me know that it would not rain again soon, in the way the birds all began singing at once, perhaps. I took my bicycle from under the tarp where it had spent the week, and rode it through the puddles as my daughter sat on the back in a child seat, an oversized helmet strapped to her chin.

"Faster, Dada, faster!" she shouted.

A symbolic ride, just enough to muddy up the virgin wheels, so our purchase of the bike rack for the van seemed like a wise investment.

"It was a good thing we rented a cabin." My wife was waiting for us beside the van, counting suitcases through the back window. "A week in a wet tent would have been awful."

We said good-bye to the campground, driving slowly down the dirt road, retracing my bicycle tracks through the puddles.

Past the rustic cabins. Past the departing campers and their collapsing tents. Past the check-in office and the new crop of campers smiling at the fresh sunshine.

Back home to the neighbors below.

"You whore!"

"You fucking dick!"

My wife opened the closet door and reached for her vacuum. "You know, the rain wasn't really so bad."

Chapter 10

𝕭

*A*UGUST CAME, and my wife still yearned for the peace of the outdoors. It was Friday, and she spotted the name of a famous horse in the morning paper.

"You're probably sick of camping," she observed cautiously.

"I love camping with you," I replied earnestly.

"It's just I hear them every night."

"I hear them too."

She folded up the sports page and handed it to me. "Yes, but you fall back to sleep. And then I hear them during the day while you're at work."

I spotted the name of the famous horse, the one she wanted to see race. "Saratoga Springs," I said. "That's a bit far."

"But it'll be cooler there," she replied. "It's been too hot here, anyway."

"We'll go tomorrow morning," I suggested. "I don't want to pitch a tent tonight in the dark."

We arrived the following day around noon. The cool mountain breezes—breezes that had drawn the wealthy out of the City in the days before airconditioning—failed to materialize.

"It's too hot here," my wife sighed. She was sitting on our blanket, squinting up at the sun with a hand shielding her eyes. "Can't we find some shade?"

"But the sun's moving that way." I pointed westward. "Soon we'll be in the shade and everyone else will be in the sun."

The sun did move, as I suspected it would, and thirty minutes later we were in the shade, where we won a few bets on the early races. But the sun continued its journey west, and soon we were no longer in the shade.

"It's too hot," my wife moaned.

Our daughter said nothing. Earlier, she had watched a horse race. I stood along the rail while she sat on my shoulders above the crowd, holding binoculars to her eyes and looking off in the wrong direction. She knew her horse's name, and cheered it on—I want to say "to victory," but I don't remember.

Later, we stopped by the little white pavilion where the famous spring bubbled with its sulfurous water. She took a drink and promptly spit it out. I bought her a bar of Häägen Dazs ice cream, which she didn't spit out. She nibbled her ice cream too slowly, chocolate dripping down around her small hand as she watched the horses parade about the paddock area, picking one for me to bet on because she thought it was crying. And I picked a horse because I thought it looked good, only to have her crying horse win and my good-looking horse come in fourth. We had done all that, but now she was tired. She was hot, too, so she said nothing as she sat on the blanket beside her mother.

My wife had stayed behind—she had not gone to the rail to

watch the race, or even to the paddock. "I'll guard our blanket," she had replied when I asked her if she wanted to come along. She watched the races on a television monitor that hung among the trees in an oversized bird feeder. A crowd formed in front of the monitor, eager to see the official finish and the payoffs, so she could no longer watch what was on the screen. The crowd cast a shadow that cooled her, but after scribbling the payoffs in their programs, they moved on, and she was once again in the sun.

"It's much too hot," she said, shaking her head slowly.

"I'm up a dollar-eighty," I replied. Reluctantly, I added, "If we leave now, at least I leave a winner."

We didn't stay to see the famous horse run—the horse that had brought us there in the first place. We left as winners instead. Only the cashier booths were too crowded, and the uncashed ticket I was holding was a show ticket worth two dollars and ten cents.

"It's awfully hot," she groaned. "Are you going to stand in that line for two dollars?"

"I've got to cash this ticket," I explained. "If I don't, I'm down thirty cents and I won't be leaving a winner."

She reached into her purse and pulled out two dollars. "Here. You're a winner." She smiled. "That means you're taking us out for dinner to celebrate."

We found a campground along the Batten Kill. It had modern toilets, but was otherwise rustic, with little more than a large grassy field with an occasional garden hose for water. It was cool, though, along the river, and that was what we needed. We took off our shoes and sat by the river's edge with our feet dangling in the water under a shady tree, and watched as a family floated by in large inner tubes.

"Let's go in, Dada."

"Sure, Pumpkin," I replied.

We returned to our tent—father and daughter—and put on

our swimsuits. I rubbed sunscreen on my daughter's egg-white arms, legs, and back.

"Don't forget the tips of her ears." My wife's voice drifted up from the riverbank, and I silently obeyed, not even questioning how she knew I had the sunscreen out.

I slipped the water wings onto my daughter's fragile arms and inflated them with shallow breaths. Then I inflated the large raft with huge breaths, growing dizzy and resting briefly in the soft grass.

We draped beach towels over our shoulders, slipped sandals onto our feet, and checked each other's legs for ticks. By the time we returned to the river, the other family was gone and the sun had dropped below the tree line, casting a cool shadow upon the riverbank.

My wife remained under the shady tree, patiently waiting for her two swimmers. In our absence, she had pulled a sweater over her shoulders. "You're not going in now?" she asked. "It's getting cold."

"We sure are," I exclaimed. I hopped in first, and our daughter jumped from the mossy bank into my arms.

"You two," my wife laughed quietly. "A couple of water bugs."

That night the moon shone with such intensity that my wife and I woke up thinking that the forest must be on fire. It was past midnight, but the children of the other campers had also been awakened by the moonlight and were playing a noisy game of softball in the grassy field beside the bathhouse. Our daughter slept on, though, lying snugly between us for warmth.

"You want me to drape some towels over the tent?" I whispered. "That will cut some of the light out."

"No," she replied. "I like it. It's surreal."

I closed my eyes and fell back asleep, but I don't think she slept for some time.

The next morning, we took the long way home—north through Vermont.

"East," she said.

"Northeast," I smiled.

We returned home to find the woman downstairs standing outside on her patio, rummaging through a stack of old dresser drawers. She looked up, pointed her finger at my wife and pulled an imaginary trigger. "Pow."

My wife shuddered.

"I'm taking you out of here," I whispered. "We'll buy a house, with our own yard, and a tree with a swing for our daughter."

"But the bankruptcy," she protested.

"I'll get us a mortgage," I promised. "You find the house you want."

We went upstairs. My wife sniffed the air. "What is that smell?"

I sniffed the air, too. "Burning chemicals," I guessed.

"No, not chemicals," she argued as she stepped toward the bathroom. "They're making drugs downstairs."

I sniffed again. "Could be. I don't really know."

"They'll blow the whole building up."

I picked up the phone, dialed a nine and a one, and was about to dial another one, then thought of the woman downstairs. I thought of her finger, and imagined it pressing against a real trigger. I thought of my wife, alone with my daughter each day—vulnerable—while I was in Boston. I thought of the strange men, driving up on motorcycles in their leather coats, climbing through the woman's window. I set the phone down.

"I'm definitely getting you out of here. We'll buy a house," I vowed again. "My father said he'll loan us the down payment."

My wife smiled, but then she thought of what I'd said. "The

down payment? We need more than the down payment. We need a mortgage, and no one will give us that."

Despite her protests, I took her house hunting. She sat rigid, her arms folded across her belly as if in a straight jacket, the seat belt and shoulder strap holding her firmly in the front seat. We parked out on the street, across from the house with the "model home" sign. The passenger door hung open, but she wouldn't get out.

"You know you're dreaming," she said.

"No, we'll get a mortgage," I replied confidently.

"But the bankruptcy." She glanced toward the house, and a sadness filled her eyes. The memory of a past home much like the one she saw saddened her.

"Find a house you like," I promised, "and I'll get us a mortgage."

She still refused to budge.

"It's a model home," I explained. "They don't care if you're really buying."

"But what if we love it," she replied solemnly. "What if we really love it, and the bank won't give us a mortgage."

"If you love it, we'll buy it." I reached in and unlatched her seat belt, then tugged her arm gently.

She resisted. "But New Hampshire is so far from Boston, and there's no train." She looked back at the child sitting peacefully in the back seat. "And I don't want you driving to work with all those idiots on the road."

"We're just getting our juices flowing," I explained. "That's all. We're not buying anything yet."

She climbed slowly from the van into the soft autumn leaves, wrapping her arms around my neck, first for support, but then to kiss me. "I love you when you're so sure of things."

As she said it, she thought of all the things she was not so sure of, and her eyes clouded over with the vacant look of a lost future.

"What's wrong?" I asked.

"Not New Hampshire," she replied softly, anxiously. "If we live so far from my sisters, after I'm gone. . ."

"But you aren't going anywhere. You're cured."

"No." She shook her head sadly. "Say it," she sighed, almost like a moan.

I knew what she wanted. Her soul—our soul—spoke to me in a whisper. Say it the way you say everything. Say it so I know that it's true.

I fixed my eyes upon her so that they would speak more than my voice. "I'll buy you a house . . ."

She smiled slightly, hearing the conviction of my voice.

". . . and we'll live there together until you're a hundred."

"You're such a dreamer," she laughed, loosening her hold on my neck and reaching into the back seat for our daughter's hand. "Come on. Let's go look at a house."

Chapter 11

WINTER RETURNED. Our second winter in Massachusetts, and it snowed more than anyone had ever seen it snow in these parts. One hundred and eight inches. Nine feet. It was a record.

"Faster, Dada, faster!"

I looked down between my legs and smiled proudly at the little girl skidding along on her plastic skis.

"Come on! Faster, Dada."

I pushed the tips of my skis together and brought the two of us to a gentle stop.

"Phooey," she replied.

"Let me rest a moment." I slowly stood up and straightened my back.

She jabbed her little plastic ski poles into the snow. "I'm not tired."

"No. You're a child," I replied. "Children never get tired."

A woman stopped along the ski trail. "How old is she?" She smiled pleasantly at the little girl standing between my skis, and eyed the bicycle helmet perched on her head like an egg.

My wife had insisted on that—the helmet. "I know you can ski," she had said. "But there are so many people on the slope who can't."

"She's two," I told the lady.

"Two-and-a-half," my daughter corrected me.

"That's how old our son is," the woman replied. "I'll have to tell my husband how you ski her along between your legs."

"It's hard on the back," I warned her. "I have to lean over and hold her up." I guessed from the woman's age that her husband was probably younger than I, so perhaps it wouldn't be hard on his back. Not yet, anyway.

My wife waited for us below, somewhere in the crowded ski lodge. A careless teenager had spilled an entire cup of hot chocolate on her new winter coat. She was mopping up the mess with a wad of paper towel when we found her.

"Did you have fun?" she asked.

"Yes!" our daughter shouted.

"I'm glad," she said. She had skied in the past—when we were first married—but the cancer had frightened her, and the treatment altered her sense of balance, giving her a feeling of falling whenever she moved too quickly.

She had been a woman of great confidence when we married, sure of how things were going to be—"I'll quit my job on the 20th of June, I'll get pregnant on the 24th. . . ."

It wasn't that way any more.

"You want to ski with us after lunch?" I asked.

She shook her head. "I don't feel like I have control over anything anymore," she sighed. "The last thing I need to do is slide around on a couple of slats of wood." She smiled. "You two go back out. You'll have more fun without me."

It snowed throughout the month of January. We sat in the window of our apartment and watched the front loader grind through the vacant parking lot. Management asked people to move their vehicles to other parking areas so ours could be cleared of snow. One vehicle remained.

The man who drove the front loader stood before the telltale snow mound and called over to the apartment manager. "What you think? There a car under here?" He rammed the dull end of a snow shovel into the pile until the hollow thud of metal told him there indeed was a car in there. Somewhere.

We watched the manager scurry through the drifting snow. He paused to pull his coat collar tight around his neck, only to have the wind betray him and blow cold blasts of snow up under the back of his coat.

"He should be wearing a hat," my wife fretted. "Why isn't he wearing a hat?"

We continued watching as he went from door to door. Finally, he came to ours.

"That your car?" he asked sharply.

I shook my head. "No."

"Know whose it is?"

I looked toward my feet, indicating the apartment below. "It hasn't moved in a month," I said. "And the registration expired sometime last summer."

"She doesn't go out?"

I shook my head again. "No."

"What does she do for food?" he asked incredulously.

"By the smell of things, she's growing fungus in her bathtub," I answered.

He sniffed the air. The foul smell from the apartment below made his nose wrinkle. "She's not answering the door. Think she might be dead?"

"No," I replied. "I just heard her shout 'fuck fuck fuck,' so she's either training her daughter in the family business, or she's out of cigarettes again."

He frowned, then quickly left our apartment. As I rejoined my wife beside the window, I could hear him pounding on the door below. We watched him wander back toward the front loader, his mission a failure, the errant car still there. He grasped his collar and ducked his head to protect his ears from the wind.

"He should wear a hat," my wife fretted again.

He stood for a moment in the blowing snow and said a few words to the driver of the front loader, then left for home.

The front loader lifted snow into arriving dump trucks, and the trucks carted it away. When there were no more dump trucks, he piled the remaining snow on the illegally parked vehicle, smiling each time he opened the bucket and an avalanche of snow rolled down over the hidden vehicle. No one saw that car again until May.

"I'm so tired of snow," my wife sighed. The front loader was gone, and she shut the blinds. "Can we go someplace warm?"

"You mean a vacation?"

"I know we should be saving our money for a house," she replied. "But no one will give us a mortgage anyway. So can't we go away?"

"We could drive to Florida," I suggested. "We could stay at your parents. That wouldn't cost too much."

"Drive?" she replied. "We'd need more than a week if we're going to drive."

"We could go for two weeks," I offered.

"What about three?" she responded cautiously. "You get three weeks, don't you?"

Use it all at once? Why not. Three weeks on the road. A leisurely spin along the entire Eastern Seaboard.

"We could visit my father, too," I added.

"And my brother," she replied. "He lives in North Carolina."

"And my aunts. They're in St. Augustine."

A plan began to take shape.

While I was at work, my wife poured over travel brochures, locating points of interest along the way. When I got home at night, she filled me in on her latest ideas.

"We don't want to spend more than five hours in the car each day." That was her rule. "With a child, I think five hours is the limit."

I plotted the course, but she made the rules.

She sat with a big map spread across her lap, running her finger from north to south, as if taking the trip in her mind. "There's nothing to see along the interstates, so avoid them whenever you can," she said, prompting me to tear up the first itinerary.

"How about the Blue Ridge Parkway?" I asked.

"Yes." She looked up from her map, her finger stuck somewhere in Florida, unwilling to return north to the snow. "That sounds nice."

"We'll have to go in April," I explained.

"Why April?" she asked impatiently. "I was hoping to leave sooner. I'm tired of winter. By April winter's gone."

"If I'm taking three weeks off from work, I have to give my boss more notice."

"I suppose the weather will be nicer then anyway. Since we're driving, that's important," she replied. "Do you think we should make reservations?"

"No. No one will be driving to Florida in April," I presumed. "At least not along the Blue Ridge Parkway."

Chapter 12

❧

I SAT AT MY DESK, looking out across the harbor as sailboats came into view, their sails hanging limp from the driving rain. I looked at my watch—an hour more, and our vacation would begin.

On the horizon, a thin yellow band. But I was facing eastward, toward yesterday's weather. I could only imagine the scene to the west—the angry dark clouds rumbling toward us like tumbleweeds, rushing in to ruin our vacation once again.

We set off that evening in a light drizzle, leaving behind an angry boss staring with confusion at his computer terminal and a depraved neighbor free to wallow in uninterrupted debauchery. The silence of our mood was highlighted by the tires spinning against the wet pavement. We were angry as we rode along, once again seeing our vacation plans fall victim to the whims of nature. We had made a mistake using up all my vacation time in one shot, to spend it in wetness and mud.

I sighed, hating the sound of the wipers slapping against the rain-soaked windshield. "Not this again."

"We've got three weeks," she replied calmly. "The sun will have to come out sooner or later."

The following day, as we entered Pennsylvania Dutch country, the sun began to break through the dark cloud cover. Determined streaks of golden sunlight fought pitched battles with the clouds, racing across the newly plowed fields, and briefly highlighting the dark stone façades of the old farm houses. My mood lightened.

"They weren't really Dutch," she explained.

"No?" I asked.

"They were German." She had been reading up for our trip.

"I see." I didn't really see. I could see mistaking Dutch for German, but not German for Dutch.

My wife had packed a bag of toys for our daughter. New toys. Just little items, but something new, nonetheless, so that the excitement of getting something new would override any boredom that the little girl might have felt from the long, lonely confinement in the seat behind us.

"Tell me when we're in Virginia, and I'll give her the troll doll." Plastics things, cheap five-and-dime store stuff, but for a two-and-a-half year old—treasures!

We skipped down the eastern seaboard—like pebbles flung from the arms of young boys to dribble across a pond. Nights we lay together on unfamiliar mattresses, their strange softness feeling odd against our travel-weary backs.

Outside our motel I heard the sounds of trucks dieseling in the parking lot, and engines straining on the nearby hills as truckers with doctored books and white pills continued their journeys late into the night.

I lay silent, staring at the ceiling, thinking. Two years this May. They said two years and she was cured, but was it two years from the start of treatment or two years from the end? There was a nine-month difference there.

Daytime, driving through the countryside, our minds flooded with the images of passing trees, women hanging laundry in the cluttered subdivisions, convicts poking trash along the highways, their guards with dark sunglasses and large shot-guns sipping coffee from a distance—we did not think of that then. But at night it would slowly creep up and stare us in the face.

"Fourteen months," she said softly.

It did not surprise me that she was awake. I was not surprised she knew what I was thinking, either. We shared the same soul. "Ten months to go then," I whispered hoarsely, rolling over and placing my arm across her shoulder, comforted that I was not alone in the darkness.

So far away—so far we had traveled, in both time and distance—and yet it was still with us.

"Ten months," she said, and patted my hand. "That's all."

We had lunch along the rim of the Skyline Drive. A quiet time of the year, and the waiter—sensing we were in no hurry—recommended we take a detour, to visit Monticello, a favorite spot of his.

Why not. With three weeks, we could take a little detour here and there.

"My boss wanted a phone number where he could reach me," I chuckled, steering the van through unfamiliar curves along a back road—a shortcut recommended to us by the hospitable waiter.

We saw an Appalachia that few people saw—homes with

tarpaper roofs, rusted cars in the front yards serving as temporary chicken coops until the price of scrap metal rebounded.

"What did you tell him?" She laughed, but she frowned also as she scrutinized the poverty around us.

"I told him we'd be traveling incognito."

"We have to be at my brother's house tonight," she reminded me. "I guess that's the only place he could reach us for sure."

"And at your parents," I added.

"But they don't really care when we show up," she replied. "They're retired."

We arrived at Monticello through quiet roads, only to find ourselves at the tail end of a huge crowd. It was the first weekend of a special exhibit.

We stood briefly in line, but my wife nudged me in the ribs. "My brother's expecting us for dinner."

I looked at my watch and saw that time would be tight. "We'll skip the mansion," I suggested. "We can just look around outside for a while."

We walked the grounds, visiting the cemetery and the slave quarters. The tour guide explained that Thomas Jefferson did own slaves, but granted them their freedom upon his death. She felt that this act was one of extreme generosity.

"If he was really generous," I suggested, "he would have freed them while he was alive and still had a use for them."

The woman gave me a dirty look, and my wife nudged me with her elbow.

I had spoken blasphemy.

Our daughter picked buttercups on the sprawling back lawn—the same lawn that Thomas Jefferson must have strolled across. Perhaps he had stopped and picked a buttercup of his own.

As a final act, we stood on our toes and peeked in the

windows of the great mansion—a mild feeling of guilt, the fleeting thought that we were snooping in on one of America's founding fathers.

We drove to her brother's and ate salmon late at night.

"Like the rich do," he laughed as he broiled the fish slowly over a gas grill.

Two years later, our daughter still remembered the visit. She remembered what Disney characters adorned the sweatshirts of her two cousins, which cousin slept in the upper bunk and which one slept in the lower one. She remembered their favorite television programs, and which one didn't like the flavor of their toothpaste.

I remembered that it took two hours to cook one fish, and we didn't eat until ten.

We left early the next morning. "We'll have to break our rule against driving on the interstate," I said. "If we want to get to my aunts' for dinner."

My wife looked up from the road map. "I suppose it's the only way."

"We'll have to drive more than five hours, too."

She sighed. "It will be easy after that, though."

The road stretched for hours across a barren pine forest— traffic coming, traffic going, but no destination anywhere to be seen. No one exiting the highway, except to fill up at the occasional gas station.

We arrived in St. Augustine and ate fish. Everywhere we went, there was fish waiting. I was a vegetarian who ate fish. When my wife and I first met, I was a vegetarian—just a vegetarian. But my wife needed a compromise. She loved to cook and needed more than vegetables to cook with, so after our wedding I agreed to eat fish.

"Daaaaahling," my eldest aunt greeted us. She was seventy and deeply wrinkled from the Arizona sun. Her skin was still tanned even though she had left the desert several years before.

"Your old aunties have been slaving away in the kitchen." She kissed my cheek and then my wife's, eyeing her closely at first for signs of death. "We know you're a vegetarian, but I thought I remembered that you ate fish."

I smiled and nodded.

"Good! Good!" She steered us through the living room and directly into the dining room. The fish was there waiting for us. "Well daaaahlings, you must be starved, driving all that way just to see your old aunties."

"We stopped along the way," I said.

"Three times," my wife added.

"Three times? I see," my aunt replied, pausing as if she found some inner meaning in what we had said. She looked downward and threw her hands up in mock surprise. "And this must be your little girl we've heard so much about!"

"Let me see! Let me see!" My other aunt ran in from the kitchen wearing an apron. It was adorned with a slogan naughtier than I remembered either aunt being in real life.

Both had been married at various times, but neither ever had children. They were always maternal—when I was a child and they visited for the holidays, it was like having an extra set of mothers in the house. Their maternal instincts had them ready to adopt any youngster that wandered through their front door.

My younger aunt looked from my daughter to me. "She looks just like your mother." She grabbed the little girl by her shoulders and twirled her around. "Doesn't she, Sis?"

"The spitting image," my eldest aunt replied.

Our daughter didn't look one bit like my mother. She looked like my wife—everyone said that.

The two aunts stood smiling at her, but the smiles slowly faded. They gradually saw what everyone else saw, and they looked at me with disappointed faces.

"She doesn't look at all like your mother," my eldest aunt sighed. "She looks like your wife."

The two seemed disappointed in the little girl, almost annoyed. They were hoping for the reincarnation of a sister they had loved dearly. Instead, they had gotten a child who was definitely becoming her own little person.

"She acts a lot like my mother did, though," I said.

"Does she?" the two replied, and smiled again.

We ate fish, then took a buggy ride around the old historic part of town. We ate dessert on the bottom of a drained swimming pool and shopped in the old Spanish Quarter.

"But daaaahlings! You can't leave us so soon," my eldest aunt wailed the following morning as she watched me pack our bags into the rear of the van.

"No, you didn't stay long enough," my younger aunt agreed.

But despite their protest, I put the van in reverse, and off we went, to my father's house, where we ate fish.

We went from there to my mother-in-law's house and ate fish.

Then we went to the Keys—where we knew no one and could eat anything we damn-well felt like eating. I ate spaghetti.

We stayed at a resort with a sea lion out back named Fernando or Ferdinand—some name or other that made me think of Spanish explorers. There were trained dolphins there, too, which I had planned to swim with, but the animal rights people shut that attraction down.

I wanted to go scuba diving, but the scuba lady told me that it would cost two hundred dollars.

"You haven't gone for over a year," she explained.

"Thirteen months," I replied.

"That's more than a year," she said. "You'll have to take my refresher course."

"I'm a creature of the sea, though."

She didn't smile. "And your equipment needs to be serviced, but I don't have time to do it, so you'll have to rent mine."

"How much are we talking about?" I asked.

"Two hundred dollars," she replied, her lips tight.

I walked next door to another marina and asked about renting a boat. Two hundred dollars again, but that was for the entire afternoon and I could take the whole family out. It also included two tanks of gas.

We went fishing in the boat and snagged small creatures on sharp hooks, then headed ashore. Only we ran out of gas, and the second tank was empty. A passing sport fisherman towed us into shore.

"That was nice of him," my wife said.

"I think it's some kind of law or something," I replied.

"It was still nice of him," she insisted.

The man at the marina swore he had filled both tanks and wouldn't reimburse me for the missing gas.

"I think there are still pirates in these waters," I told my wife.

"I know there are pirates, but they live on land now." She showed me the receipt for a T-shirt she had bought. Forty dollars.

"Forty dollars for a T-shirt?" I gasped.

"I didn't check the charge slip until I was leaving the shop," she explained. "When I went back and asked him about it, he said it was twenty dollars extra for the decal."

"Twenty dollars for a decal?"

The pirates had indeed become landlubbers.

I took my daughter swimming in the hotel pool. A woman floated by, slowly kicking her feet and moving her arms. My daughter stared at her, then stared at me. "Hey! Mommies can swim!"

"Some mommies can swim," I explained.

Hers didn't, though. Perhaps it was the short summers of northern New Hampshire, or perhaps it was the polluted waters—the paper mills—of the local rivers where she had grown up. Whatever the cause, my wife had never developed a fondness for swimming. After her operations and her scars, she wasn't fond of wearing bathing suits. Our daughter had never seen her mommy in the water. She never asked why, and we never mentioned it. In her young mind, she developed a belief that daddies swam and mommies did not. It was as simple as that.

"Some mommies swim," I said. "But yours doesn't."

In the evenings, the dolphins put on a show in the hotel's man–made lagoon. In return, they were given their supper. Our final night, we watched the last dolphin leap far into the air, an elegant dark creature silhouetted against the red sunset.

We headed north, moving slower than on the trip south as if the map's upward tilt were holding us back. We drove along the Gulf Coast, breaking our rule and using the interstate, traveling too far from the beach to even smell the salt air. Then we crossed the panhandle and entered Georgia as night fell.

It began to rain. It hadn't rained since the start of the trip. It hadn't even been cloudy. We'd had good luck—no rain, plenty of fish, hospitable relatives.

No cancer.

Two years. Two years, and she was considered cured. Two years, and her doctor would pull the portacath from her chest and declare her saved. I lay awake nights listening to her breathe, thinking that each night her breath sounded stronger than the night before.

We were having good luck. No rain, no cancer.

But then it started to rain, and I thought our good luck had given out.

We felt the thunder, shaking us in the middle of the night

from our restless sleep. Come morning, my wife sat in the silent darkness of the motel as I struggled to brushed my teeth. The power was out.

"No hot water, either," I called from the small bathroom.

"We were going to Callaway Gardens today," she sighed, a sense of defeat in the way she said it. We had swung this far west so she could visit the famous gardens—her only request. Now rain had come.

"We'll stay another day," I offered. "It might clear up tomorrow."

"No, that's okay," she replied, resignation hanging on each word like a great sadness. "We don't know how long the rain will last. Let's keep moving."

I walked through the grayness of the room and draped my arms over her shoulders. "We can drive through the gardens anyway," I suggested. "You can see the flowers from the van."

I could feel her nod her head, but it was a slow, sad nod. "There's an arboretum there too," she said as I kissed her soft hair. "We can tour that, I suppose."

We headed toward Atlanta, so close to Alabama that I couldn't pass it by.

"We've never been to Alabama," I reminded her.

"It's almost eleven," my wife observed. "If you'd like to see Alabama, we could go there for lunch."

We crossed the Chattahoochee river, running thick and brown like a never-ending supply of chocolate milk, and entered Alabama, unwittingly entering a new time zone where it was still ten o'clock and the restaurants were closed, or those that were open were serving eggs and grits.

"I don't think I want eggs for lunch," I said, frowning.

"Neither do I," my wife agreed heartily. "And definitely not grits."

We crossed back over the river into Georgia—to the eastern time zone where burgers and french fries were being served.

We spent less than five minutes in Alabama, but I still counted it, adding it to the mental list of states we had visited.

"Keep going," she ordered. "We'll find someplace to eat at Callaway Gardens."

Around noon, we saw the gates to the garden. I looked across the vast lawns of the nearby golf course and saw movement upon the grass—shadows. "The clouds are breaking up," I observed cautiously.

She saw it, too. A faint smile came to her face. Our luck was returning. Maybe after lunch the sun would be out. And maybe after two years her cancer would be cured.

The sun did not shine, though, except for an occasional tease. But it didn't rain either. After lunch, we toured the gardens, lone tourists among the dripping rhododendrons.

The following day, we entered the Great Smoky Mountains. The sun shone with a convincing brilliance that told us that Callaway Gardens had been a fluke.

I parked outside a motel, and she stepped from the van into bright sunlight. "Only one night here?" she asked, looking quickly toward the scratch pad that held our itinerary.

I looked around, at the mountains, the sunshine. I looked in the back seat at the sleeping child and beside the van at the tired woman.

"We can stay longer if you like," I suggested. "We'll skip Gettysburg."

"Let's then," she said.

We stayed three days, and panned for gems while our daughter slept in her car seat, placed under the shade of a nearby tree. We hiked under a sky of uninterrupted blue and felt the early heat as we searched for souvenirs in Cherokee. The crowds had not come yet—it was still April. Or had we traveled into May by then?

We went to the Indian museum and went to Indian stores and bought Indian crafts because my wife had learned the history of the Cherokee and knew that we owed them something.

"You're part Indian, though," I reminded her.

"Not much," she replied, fingering a dream catcher in the little museum shop. "One-sixteenth, maybe."

"That might be enough to own a casino," I said.

"I'm Norwegian, mostly," she explained.

"I don't think the Norwegians ever stole land from the Indians." I flipped over a tom–tom expecting to see "Made in Mexico," but found hand–carved initials. Quality.

"In North Dakota they did."

"Yes," I laughed. "But nobody really wanted to live in North Dakota, anyway."

She selected a small basket and paid the Indian lady who stood stoically behind the counter.

From Cherokee we drove west to Dollyland, go-carts, and Ferris wheels; Honky Tonk Tennessee where I bought fireworks and stashed them in the attic once we got home because my wife wouldn't let me shoot them off.

"It's against the law," she explained.

"Lots of things are against the law," I replied.

We stopped for gas in a small town in northern Tennessee. A little girl smiled at me and waved enthusiastically. I waved back.

A woman sat beside the cash register in an aluminum lawn chair. "Ignore him. The man's a snake," she said to the child.

I didn't think it was meant as a compliment. I thought it had something to do with our Massachusetts license plate and the Civil War, and something to do with them living out too far in the country.

We toured the farmlands of Virginia, traveling as far as the Cumberland Gap. Daniel Boone! History, I told my wife, but it was really an excuse to extend the trip, to keep driving, ride faster and faster until our troubles could no longer keep up.

Then we swung back east, up the Shenandoah Valley, and re-entered the states we were familiar with.

"Don't get too far east," my wife warned. "We don't want to go through New Jersey."

"I grew up in New Jersey," I replied defensively.

"Yes, well then you've seen enough of it."

We continued north through Pennsylvania, east across New York, and entered Connecticut. And there it was.

Three thousand miles. Perhaps it was four thousand. And after all that distance, the road that traveled homeward brought us within a quarter mile of that place. Our former home.

"Do you want to see it?" I asked.

"No, I don't want to see it," she replied. "Do you?"

"No. I don't want to see it."

But we had to see it, passing so close that the vision of our lives reflected vaguely across the highway like waves of heat on a steamy summer day. Off in the distance, a mirage, our first home. We were wed there. Our daughter was conceived there.

To avoid looking. . .

But we couldn't avoid looking, any more than the most well-mannered, respectable traveler could avoid looking—just a peek—as he passed the scene of a horrific automobile accident, glancing sideways out the car window without actually turning his head, seeing just enough. No, I didn't really look. I'm not one of those—a rubbernecker, he'd claim to himself as he shuddered at the sight of so much blood.

That was what it was like for us. We didn't want to go back, but we had to, drawn by a distinct desire to see if it was all true, if it had really happened at all, or was just one of those bad dreams.

Pinch me, and it will end.

The foreclosure sign was gone, no longer advertising failure: come see the home of the big flop family! That was good.

The fence was gone, too, and that was sad. It was built stick by stick during one of those early springs. The weather turned unseasonably warm, and my wife lounged in the hammock, saying, "I know it's going to be a girl, but does that make you sad?"

"A girl? No, I'd love a girl." A girl, a child that would cuddle with her father, keep cuddling long after a son had gone off to cuddle with his girlfriend.

I designed the fence myself and built it by hand. "Do you think the lattice should be white?"

"Yellow," my wife replied as she lay in the hammock stroking her tummy.

"Then brown for the tongue and groove?"

"Of course," she replied. "And the gate, too."

I dug the post holes by hand. Rent an auger, I was told, but the auger down at the hardware store was a two-man tool, and we were a man and a woman, and almost with a child.

But the fence was gone. It required maintenance, and that can be a hard word for some people to swallow. Tear it down and wave hello to the neighbors. Live life the easy way.

Our dog was gone, too. Fenced in amongst the prettiest flowers we'd ever grown, her puppy ways told her to yank up those snapdragons and shake them until they were dead.

"She's digging up the garden again."

"Bad dog. Bad bad doggie."

She'd wag her tail and yank up one more snapdragon—shake it right under my nose—just to let me know she understood completely what I was saying.

She was gone, too, along with the fence.

The rock garden was also gone. One rock remained. Someone had painted it white and yanked out the flowers more efficiently than our dog ever could, then planted green crab grass all around. There the rock sat, a big white eyeball lying in the middle of the yard.

Everything was gone.

The house was still there, but it was made of vinyl and glue and staples. It was never part of us. We were hardier than that. We belonged in a house of oak and slate, planted firmly on a massive granite foundation.

"Was there a sidewalk?" she asked as we left the old neighborhood and drove back toward the interstate.

"I didn't notice."

How could I not have noticed? We fought the town for two years, trying to get them to build the sidewalks that we had already paid for.

But so much was missing—the fence, the gardens, the dog—us. Who could fault me for not noticing what was now there?

"We shouldn't have gone back there," my wife sighed. "It made me sad."

"You knew it would make you sad," I replied. "That's why we had to go back."

Chapter 13

☙

*S*HE FOUND HER HOUSE.

The real estate agent drove us there, and we sat before it in his car with the engine idling. We stared up into the welcoming eyes of the aging Queen Anne Victorian.

"We were looking for something a bit less extravagant," I remarked.

"It's lovely," my wife gasped.

"It belongs to you," the real estate agent replied.

Two days together with him and he knew. Remarkable, but he knew. Oak, mahogany, solid wood doors. A granite foundation! We had never told him, but he knew.

He had driven us through the new neighborhoods of the town—the prestigious addresses. We nodded our heads and said "very nice," but he knew the truth and drove us there.

"Can we go inside?" she asked.

"Of course," he replied. "It's your house."

"We could never afford it," she sighed.

"Make an offer." It will be yours, his voice seemed to say.

"Oh, a stained glass window!" She stepped into the foyer and stared about at the carved mahogany staircase. She pointed up the staircase toward the center of the window. "A bluebird!" She grabbed my hand and pulled me closer. "My grandmother always said a bird in the house was bad luck, but I think it's pretty."

The owner was preparing dinner in the kitchen. The smell of sautéed garlic lingered in every room. My wife let the aroma guide her to its source.

"Oh, look at the kitchen." She stood before the center island and ran her fingers across its smooth almond-colored surface.

The owner listened proudly as we strolled through the house and remarked on the same features he would have remarked on. The crown molding, the beautiful mirrored fireplace, the glass door knobs. There was a coffered ceiling in the master bedroom, not original to the house, but an addition set in place by a transient carpenter. Yellow pine floors, real plaster walls. Authentic oil light fixtures with amber glass and burnished brass fittings.

We didn't ask about the square footage—one could see it was more than enough house for three. We didn't ask about the number of bathrooms. That was not important.

The owner knew, too. Yes, this house was ours, just as it had been his before us; just as he had never asked about square footage or about bathrooms, but had stared at the bluebird in the stained glass window.

"A swing!" our daughter shouted.

No, there wasn't a swing. But there was a tree with a limb growing parallel to the ground, and the grass scrubbed away underneath, the earth packed hard by the feet of an earlier generation of children now grown and off at college. There was no swing now, but there had been—the bits of dangling rope betrayed that—and there would be again, for the house belonged to us. The three of us. For a hundred years.

"Seven years," the banker stated. "Seven years until I can give you a mortgage."

I sat before the massive desk and stared in disbelief. "Seven years?"

"Yes," he growled. "You've got to wait seven years after bankruptcy for your credit to be restored." He pulled unrelated paperwork from a pile, eager to dismiss me.

"Thank you," I said, then left. Thank you, but you must be wrong, for, you see, the house is waiting for us now.

Seven years. Rapists get rehabilitated quicker than that.

"Seven years," they all growled, at eight different banks.

"Well, they're wrong," the man at bank number nine told me, looking out over the top of his glasses.

"They're wrong?" I straightened up in the chair, regaining the posture my past failures had destroyed.

He took a manual out from under his desk and thumbed far into it. "Somewhere, somewhere." Past the well-worn spots that he had often visited and back into the stiff pages where few fingers had ever ventured.

He pushed his glasses closer to his face and squinted. "Two years." He set the heavy tome down with a thud and spun it so I could see. "If the bankruptcy was due to events outside your control, Fannie Mae guidelines say you qualify two years after the discharge."

"It's been over a year," I explained. "But not two."

"Hmm." He picked the book up again and continued reading, moving his finger slowly down the page. His finger stopped.

"One year," he said.

"One year?" I asked, hope filling my voice.

"If the bankruptcy was the result of a medical emergency, then you can qualify for a mortgage after one year." He removed his glasses and stuffed them in his breast pocket.

I stayed behind as the other passengers jostled their way from the train. They shuffled down the platform, a lump of humanity, poking one another with umbrellas, stepping on the heels of their fellow commuters. The conductor paused briefly beside my seat then continued on, satisfied that I was aware we were in the station. A strange feeling passed through my mind, a little piece of euphoria. I sat perfectly still hoping to recapture it, to trap it and hold it, examine it and understand it so that I could recall the feeling over and over again like a junkie reaching for that incredible high.

But it was gone.

I walked down Canal Street, looking past the tops of buildings, beyond the sky, to where my thoughts became real, asking myself, "What was it, what was it, what was it?"

It was happiness—uninhibited happiness. Not the bittersweet happiness of hearing our daughter read "cat" for the very first time, her mother smiling by her side as I looked on, knowing that my wife might not be there for her later. This was unbridled happiness.

It had been two years since the day my wife had been told. Two years, and my mind was beginning to break free from the storm that brewed within it.

"Honey." I called my wife from work. "The bank's approving our loan today."

"The banks aren't open yet," she replied cautiously. "How could you know?"

"I just know."

I hung up the phone and waited anxiously. The feeling I'd had on the train was gone, that little snip of euphoria. But it had been replaced by a vague sense of optimism. I waited until nine o'clock, then sat drumming my fingers on a mouse pad, waiting a few eternal minutes more so the man at the bank could get his coffee, hoping that would put him in a better mood. Then I phoned.

"Have we been approved?" I anxiously asked.

"No," he said. "I tried, but my boss said no." I could hear him fumbling with his glasses.

"But it's been a year, and it was a medical emergency, and we have the down payment, and we qualify, and we did everything you asked," I cried. "And the house is waiting for us."

And if I tell my wife, she'll cry, and she's cried enough already.

"My boss said no. I'm sorry," he replied sympathetically. "I have a friend, though. He works at a different bank, with a different boss, and he wants to help." He gave me the friend's phone number.

I called, and the friend didn't say no.

The friend's boss didn't say no, either. He said, "I'm scared." The rule was there in black and white—one year. Far back in the book perhaps, in pages unfamiliar to most, but it was there nonetheless. No one had ever used the rule, though, which frightened him.

"My boss wants me to call Washington first," the friend told me. "He wants me to get Fannie Mae's opinion about their rule."

He called Washington. I drummed mouse pads, nervously marking time. He asked Fannie Mae about the rule, but they were scared, too. The rule was there, but no one had ever used it. It was like test driving a rocket ship for the first time, and it frightened them.

"It's a good loan," the friend told Washington. "They're good people."

But they were scared in Washington, too, so they told him to decide.

The friend's boss wouldn't make the decision. "I'm not sticking my neck out," he told the friend. "If I have to make the decision, I'll say no."

"Then let me make the decision," the friend pleaded. "These are good people. This is a good loan. Let me decide."

The boss thought about it. "Yes, you decide."

The friend decided. He stuck his neck out, and the house was ours.

Chapter 14

❧

"It looks sort of silly without furniture," my wife commented as she stared at the lone lamp sitting in the front parlor.

The room was a bit time–worn, but it was still a fine example of Victorian architecture. Middle class architecture—that's what we had been told. Two large doorways opened into the parlor, one from the front foyer and the other from the dining room. The two doorways had originally held pocket doors—that was obvious from the thickness of the walls—but the doors themselves had been lost to modernization.

The heights of the walls were decorated with the original gold–leaf molding, and high mahogany baseboards hugged the bottom. The floors were of yellow pine polished to a high gloss. It was not the pine of today, soft and squishy, grown too quickly to flood the coffers of the lumber companies. It was the pine of an earlier, more patient era—hard, durable, unblemished, except for an occasional mark from another era, when women tottered about the room precariously perched upon the spikes of high-heeled shoes.

The ceilings were high by current standards and coated with real plaster. Horse hair had been mixed with the plaster for added strength. The ceiling was cracked with age, but the horse hair had done its job, keeping the plaster in place long after the horse had been evicted from the barn in favor of an automobile.

An oil lamp hung from the center of the ceiling. It was not original to the house—the following year, I would find the gas pipes in the ceiling, suggesting that when the house was built, it had been quite modern for its time and equipped with gas lights.

But with all these features, the most startling thing was that, except for a floor lamp, the room was empty.

"We're starting over," I replied. "Starting from scratch. The room should be empty."

"None of our old furniture would have worked anyway," she said. "Too modern." She took my hand and led me into the foyer, to stand together before the stained glass window and view the bluebird. "It's all ours now," she sighed.

"Yes." I squeezed her hand gently.

"I don't know how you did it."

"You did it," I replied. "By making me love you so."

The bluebird seemed to flutter its wings, an illusion created by a birch tree swaying in the breeze behind it. I looked at my wife and smiled. Her grandmother had told her a bird in the house was bad luck, but I didn't believe it.

"It feels like this house is truly ours," she said.

"It is," I replied sarcastically. "We just bought it."

"Not in that way." She walked into the dining room, and I

followed. "It's like we've lived here before. I knew each of the rooms before I even saw them."

"Perhaps we were Victorian lovers in a previous life."

She smiled at the idea. "Come. Sit with me." She looked about as I pulled a chair up next to hers. "We'll keep the dining room furniture for now. It's modern, but I think it works."

The living room furniture was Scandinavian. It didn't work, but it would have to do for awhile.

"An apple!" our daughter shouted, holding one up as she came from outside, where she had been looking for a spot for her swing.

The swing was easy. The rotted ends of two ropes still hung from the limb of an old sugar maple, the spot chosen decades before and still used on windy days by ghost children. Nature had chosen the spot—it had sent a tree limb out that was perfect for a swing. Nature knew where the swing should go too—outside the kitchen window where a careful mother busily slathering peanut butter between two slices of bread could still watch her child play.

The swing was easy, but our daughter went searching for other spots that adults couldn't see. A small shrub—no, a secret garden. Just a berry bush—no, a Christmas tree already decorated. A rock—the Kuala Mountains! She went exploring and found her own apple tree, with one lone apple waiting there for her, hanging at just the right height for her reach. The tree knew that we were coming home.

My wife smiled at our daughter. "Wash it first," she said as she watched the little girl rub the apple against her shirt. Then she looked again at the parlor—empty, except for the lone floor lamp. "Perhaps the JC Penny catalog will have some inexpensive chairs in it."

"And a coffee table," I agreed, leading her back to the living room and the Scandinavian-style sofa.

Chapter 15

꙳

Autumn snuck in before we had unpacked the last of the boxes.

"I know I have a one–quart sauce pan," my wife mused. "But I can't find it anywhere."

We found it as Halloween approached. It had been tossed into the box marked COSTUMES, a hurried reaction in the panic of moving.

"I remember now," I explained. "I thought the wigs would keep it from getting dented."

"Men are so strange."

Outside, the sugar maples that lined the sidewalk were slowly losing their leaves. Two sickly ones lost their leaves quickly, but the others put on a brilliant red-orange display that lingered for weeks.

My wife and I raked half the fallen leaves on a sunny but cool Saturday morning. Autumn, and everything had turned crisp—the leaves were crisp, the morning air was crisp, even the elongated shadows we cast were crisp. We raked the leaves into tidy piles, then stuffed them into jumbo paper bags before our daughter could scatter them across the lawn as she practiced dance steps of her own invention.

"Really, Dada. We do a leaf dance in school," she said with her impish grin, knowing that she wasn't going to fool me. "Really. We do!"

"You're a corn dog," I replied as I watched her hop from one leaf to the next, singing a little la-la song about leaf fairies and acorns—something she was making up as she went along.

She was three and started dancing school that September, the first privilege that the young child was to gain by virtue of age alone. Her cousins had come to her birthday party and helped her blow out the candles, then invited her into the sorority of the dancing cousins—five little dancing girls, one for each finger, a true handful.

We went inside for lunch while our daughter stayed outside to throw sticks for Bobo, her invisible dog.

"Don't scatter those leaves, you two," I yelled through an open window.

"It was Bobo," she explained. "Bad Bobo. No more sticks for you."

"Be nice to Bobo," I replied. "He's just a puppy." I joined my wife in the kitchen and chuckled slightly as I grabbed her softly by her shoulders. She winced.

"Hurt yourself?" I asked.

"Uh huh," she moaned. "Feels like I broke it."

"Rest then," I said. "I'll finish the raking."

"I'm sorry. I'm not much of a wife."

I kissed her hair. "You're a perfect wife. You're just not much of a farm hand."

The next morning, her shoulder was no better.

"You really strained it good," I said. I gently massaged her neck and shoulder as we stood together in the kitchen, gathering breakfast inspiration by staring into the refrigerator.

"Can I go outside with Bobo?" our daughter interrupted.

"Go, go," I said, too impatiently. I rubbed my wife's shoulder some more. "I'll work it out. It's just a tired muscle."

"No," my wife whispered. "It's come back."

"No," I argued. "Your last blood test was normal. Your tumor marker was normal. You just strained it."

It couldn't be back. She was cured.

But her shoulder didn't get better.

"The x–ray does show something odd." Her doctor clipped the sheet of black plastic into the view box and squinted at the vague image of her shoulder. "It doesn't look like cancer, though."

A CAT scan would show more than an x–ray, he told us. He set up an appointment for the following morning.

That night, we sat together in our bed, propped up by half a dozen pillows. I gently rubbed her breasts, imagining I had healing powers. Kill! Seek out and kill cancer cells! I sent commands through my fingertips as my hands swept toward her aching shoulder.

Her doctor called the following evening with the radiologist's report. "The CAT scan also shows something," he explained. "It doesn't look quite like cancer, though." He ordered a biopsy, the only way to tell for sure.

She lay that night across our bed as I rubbed lotion on her back, softly touching those parts that were sore.

"I don't know why they didn't do a biopsy first off," she complained. "Instead, they kept us worrying for a week."

"If it's cancer, though. . ."

"If it's cancer, then I know what it is and what I have to do," she replied briskly. "It's the waiting that's hard."

The biopsy needle was jabbed, and my wife was right. The cancer was back—in the bones this time. The cancer was back, and our brief period of personal warmth and sunshine was coming to an end just as the leaves of the maples fell to the ground bringing winter to all.

We sat upon our bed once more. This time she avoided the pillows and lay her head directly against my shoulder, sobbing gently.

I stroked her hair, but said nothing.

"I was wrong," she cried. "It's not the waiting that's hard. It's the knowing."

Chapter 16

꒰ꕥ꒱

I HELD HER ELBOW as we entered the doctor's office, and set her in a wooden armchair surrounded by family pictures—pictures of the doctor's happy, smiling children and his healthy wife. I looked from the pictures to my wife, and finally to the doctor. "What can you do for us?" I asked.

He listed the options. But we all knew what was called for, and when he finally said it, we looked to each other and smiled grimly. A bone marrow transplant.

That was her best chance, he explained. They would harvest bone marrow from her blood and save it, then give her a fatally therapeutic dose of drugs—fatal because it would kill the bone marrow that remained in her body, therapeutic because it would also kill the cancer. Then when everything was dead, they would inject the harvested bone marrow back into her bloodstream and it would start growing in her hollow bones. Simple. Oh—and she'd have to stay in a hospital bubble-room for a month until the bone marrow grew back because it's the marrow that fights disease. And yes—there was a chance the bone marrow wouldn't grow back, and an infection would kill her.

"Does your daughter go to school?" her doctor asked.

"No. She's only three," my wife replied.

"Good. School kids bring home a lot of infections."

We knew what to expect. My wife read all the medical literature she could find, while I read the insurance literature. Our bases were covered—we sat with an air of composure in the waiting room outside the transplant team's office. In a darkened corner, a frail couple huddled under a shawl like a scene from Ellis Island—refugees in a strange land.

Their shell–shocked eyes looked straight through me. I looked away, at the coffee table before me and saw a book— a large book with beautiful color photos, like a coffee table book, except it was titled *Histiocytosis*. I stared at the title— *Histiocytosis*, not a coffee table book at all.

I shook my head.

My mother died of histiocytosis. She had it for many months, only she never knew it. The doctors didn't know she was dying because their machines didn't tell them. She knew she was dying, but she didn't know why. After she died, the doctors did an autopsy, and then they knew, but of course, it was too late.

"It's very difficult to diagnose," her doctors explained. "And very rare."

We were naïve and trusted them. I told people who asked that my mother had died of something very rare and extremely hard to diagnose, yet here I was in the transplant team's waiting room looking at an entire coffee table book about that supposedly rare disease.

I had learned from my mother's mistake. She had died so that my wife could live. She had stayed in Connecticut, where the doctors couldn't help her. I learned from that—I learned that I should bring my wife to Boston.

An orderly poked his head into the waiting room. He saw the frail couple and looked quickly away. He saw us and smiled slightly.

"Come," he beckoned.

We entered a stark conference room. Two doctors joined us. One was older and distant, while the other was young and personable—he hadn't lost any patients yet. In time, he would be older and distant, too, I imagined.

They explained the protocol. My wife would be treated with conventional chemotherapy—Taxol—to measure its effectiveness. No point in doing high dose chemo if low dose did nothing. That was the theory.

"But wouldn't a low dose give the cancer a chance to build up immunity to the drugs?" I asked. "Shouldn't we just sneak in and zap it with the high dose?" I was thinking of fruit flies and pesticides.

"That is a valid theory. We don't really know," the older doctor replied. "But we have to show your insurance company that chemotherapy is effective before they'll authorize the treatment."

The insurance company. That was my department, so I listened closely.

"Your doctor has you on hormones?" the older doctor asked. "Leuprolide?"

"Yes," my wife answered. "He stopped the tamoxifen."

"Okay. Stay with that until we can get the Taxol."

It was three months before they got the Taxol. Originally it came from tree bark, gathered in the west by scavengers, salvaged during clear–cutting by lumber mills. Car loads of bark boiled down to one dose. Now there was a synthetic version. Scientists said it was identical to the natural kind, but how would they know? How could they be sure there wasn't something science couldn't see, something that didn't show up, but was there nonetheless?

We waited for three months, while my wife's treatment consisted of a hormone that we had little faith in. But then they started the Taxol, and my wife dusted off her wig.

She didn't even wait for her hair to fall out. She believed them when they told her there would be heavy hair loss. That evening, when we got home from her first treatment, she handed me the sewing scissors.

"Cut it off."

"I can't," I replied sadly. I held the scissors limply in my hand.

"Don't be a baby," she scolded. "You won't hurt me."

"It's not that," I sighed. "I just can't do it. It'll make you unhappy."

She grabbed the scissors from my hand and began chopping blindly at the side of her head.

I worried she'd chop an ear off, so I relented. "How short?"

"Cut it all off," she demanded.

And so I did.

She didn't go out—it was winter anyway, but her absence was curious enough to our neighbors. We saw them as they strolled past the house too frequently and too slowly, their eyes darting discreetly toward our windows.

"Close the curtains, please," my wife insisted. "They're staring in." She tightened her bandanna. She wouldn't wear the wig in the house—it was too itchy—but she had a collection of bandannas that she made full use of when I was home. When she was alone—alone meaning our daughter and her— she wore nothing on her head.

She went each month for her Taxol, getting sicker and sicker with each treatment, fighting desperately to make it to the end. Spring arrived. Her legs were too weak to carry her, so I set her in a wheelchair. I rolled her into the hospital, bald headed, nauseous, her mouth too sore to talk, where they lay her under the bone scanner and checked the results.

The cancer had spread.

"They're not going to let me in the program," she cried. We were once again sitting in the transplant team's waiting room.

A woman huddled nearby with a child. I looked over, thinking to myself, "Not the child. Please not the child."

We could hear the two doctors in the next room consulting with the radiologist. "The cancer spread," someone said.

"No effect," another replied.

"Her only chance." The young doctor, I assumed. He was still a virgin—yet to lose a patient, and still believed in his power to heal.

"It spread," my wife moaned.

"Of course it spread," I replied angrily. "They didn't treat you for three months—except with Leuprolide, and we knew that wouldn't work." I spoke loudly, responding to my wife, but really responding to the doctors. If I could hear them, they could hear me. I didn't want a confrontation—the wall that separated us would prevent that—but merely some input. If they heard what I said—heard it from a distance, from another room, perhaps feeling that the words drifted down to them from up above—they could adopt my view as their own without admitting openly that it came from me, a non-doctor. "They should have done a bone scan just before the Taxol, not just before the Leuprolide. Now we don't know if the cancer spread in the three months before the Taxol or the three months during the Taxol."

"They won't let me in the program." She stared at me oddly, not understanding why I was being so loud.

"They have to let you in," I shouted. "They screwed up, and now they have to give you the benefit of the doubt."

"But the Taxol didn't work."

The two transplant doctors walked the radiologist from the conference room. The younger doctor was smiling as the older one signaled for us to join them. We settled into the uncomfortable plastic chairs, and the older doctor proceeded to explain the situation.

"We compared the bone scan from before the Taxol with the bone scan from after the Taxol, and it shows that the cancer had spread."

"But . . ." I began.

He held up his hand. "However, the first bone scan was taken three months before the Taxol began."

My wife slowly turned her eyes toward me, and I smiled back.

I have powers, see? Mind control, I said to her with my smile.

"So we can't tell whether or not the Taxol worked." He closed his folder. "The only fair thing we can do is let you into the program." The two doctors stood up. They didn't smile, but they seemed pleased with what they were saying, even if they were speaking my words and not their own. "The social worker will be in shortly to explain everything to you."

Early Spring. We waited for my wife to be admitted into the bone marrow transplant program.

While we waited, I decided to paint the house. "Should I?"

"Sure," she replied as she sat on our porch reading a medical journal.

It had been a white house when we bought it, but white was so . . . white. The Victorians would never have lived in a white house.

"I really am going to paint it," I warned her.

"Go ahead," she replied. "It's our house. You can paint it if you want."

I went to the local paint store and got a booklet of paint samples. Historic colors, they called it.

"How about these four colors?" my wife asked as she viewed the booklet of paint chips, the medical journal forgotten on the floor.

"Which one?" I asked.

"All of them."

All of them. The house was a Queen Anne Victorian—peaks and gables, an assortment of shingles, dentils, spindles, clapboard. A plethora of nineteenth-century architectural items. Porches with turned posts. Bay windows. She showed me a book of houses from San Francisco and Cape May.

"Like these," she explained. "Painted Ladies, they call them."

Okay. A painted lady it is.

The color scheme took form. I divided the house into two large fields, sage above and tan below. The small dentils between the first and second story—between the sage and the tan—would be dark brown with a cream background. Along the eaves, the large dentils would reverse the scheme—cream with a dark brown background.

"What about the windows?" my wife asked as she stood in the sunshine looking up at the house.

"The vertical lines should be cream. Horizontal lines should be dark brown, as a general rule," I explained. "Anything else I come across, I'll just wing it."

I did a strip in the back corner from the eaves to the foundation, four feet wide, just enough to get an idea.

"What do you think?" I asked as I stepped back to admire my work.

She stood toward the rear of the driveway and squinted up at my work in the afternoon light. "I like the white better." She stared at me, then laughed. "No. I think that's it."

"You think?" I asked.

"Go for it," she replied.

While I painted, she waited, standing naked against the disease. Her only defense was the continued use of Leuprolide—already proven ineffective.

The cold wind blew. Spring was still young. I climbed down from the ladder and put my paint brush away. I'd try again tomorrow.

She sat in the living room, teaching our daughter how to tie her shoes. I watched silently, then joined them on the sofa.

The television played, but no one watched.

"What are you thinking about?" she asked.

She could tell when I was deep in thought. I tried to fool her by staring at the television, nodding my head as the newscaster droned on like I was agreeing with something he said, but she knew.

"Nero," I replied.

I couldn't help it. When I wasn't thinking about paint, I was thinking about Nero and his fiddle. I should have been thinking about my wife and trying to understand what she felt. I felt guilty, sitting there deep in my own thoughts, when I should have been thinking about my wife, but all I could think of was ancient Rome and Nero and his damn fiddle.

She understood, though—she saw that in reality I was thinking of her. "I could be dead before they do anything," she sneered.

"The insurance company would like that," I replied.

"But what do I need all these tests for?" she complained. "I mean, really. A heart test? So if my heart's weak, they're going to let me die of cancer instead of risking a heart attack? That doesn't make any sense."

"I think the government must be involved in there somewhere," I replied.

Her hair began to grow back. Slowly.

"It's coming in red this time." She stood before a full length mirror. The previous owner had hung it in the bathroom to make the small room appear large.

"And straight," I added as I stood beside her. I could have easily looked directly at her hair, but instead I viewed it in the bathroom mirror as she did.

"It is straight." She ran her fingers through it. "It's still short. Maybe it'll curl when it gets longer."

We were dressing up. She hadn't been out of the house—other than for medical reasons—for months, but our daughter's dance recital was that afternoon. She was going to be a firefly and dance to "This Little Light Of Mine."

The auditorium lights dimmed, the curtain rose, and eight little girls in white tutus and gold-and-white veils studded with blinking lights shuffled unsurely onto the stage. The music started, and our daughter took her first step.

The other girls looked right, then left. Ah, there she is. Our leader. The others' confidence grew as they followed our daughter's example. She knew the words, she knew the steps. I sat in the darkness and tears formed in my eyes, tears for my wife, that she had lived to see this. Not three months as the first doctor had said—she had lived three years and had seen her daughter dance.

The song ended too soon. She had known the words and the steps. She remembered to touch her lips and to throw the crowd a kiss.

But then she remembered what her mother had said—"You've got lipstick on, so don't touch your lips."

She shook her hands like they were covered with ants, and hopped on one foot before the audience. "Oh! My mommy told me not to touch my lips!"

Everyone laughed. We laughed, too.

"But, dear," my wife explained as we drove home in the car. "They were laughing with you, not at you."

"But why? Wasn't I good?"

"You were wonderful," she replied. "But tomorrow don't worry about your lips."

Yes. It was the dress rehearsal, and tomorrow we could watch her dance again, and I would cry again. She would do it without the ad-lib, and afterward, her aunts would fill her little arms with flowers.

I painted too much. I painted after work and on weekends. I painted while we watched television, dashing outside when an advertisement came on, then dashing back in, too late to see the start of the show, pestering my wife to fill in the missing details.

"Where are you?" My wife could smell the fish cooking. She could see the smoke rising from the grill. But where was the chef?

"I'm up here, honey."

She looked up and saw me on the ladder, the spatula traded in for a paint brush. "You're watching the fish, aren't you?"

"I've got the egg timer on," I called down.

"You don't have your old clothes on," she observed. "You'll get paint on your good shorts."

"I'll be careful."

Painting. Stealing moments from my wife and from my daughter. Precious moments. Then one Saturday morning my daughter stood at the bottom of the ladder looking up at me.

"Won't you ever play with me again?" she asked.

I looked down and saw the young face. I saw a face that would not stay young forever. But the paint, that would always be there, never-changing buckets of latex goo. I climbed down the ladder and set my brushes in a bucket of warm water. "What should we play?"

"Baseball!" she exclaimed.

So we did. We played using odd rules of our own invention. After that, I didn't paint anymore when the others were awake. Instead I got up at four-thirty each morning—well before my wife and daughter awoke—sipping my coffee on the front porch, rocking back and forth slowly in my green rocking chair. Casually, I planned my morning's work, and when the sun had risen enough for me to see, I would paint.

Chapter 17

❧

"**W**HERE'S THE DOCTOR?" I asked the receptionist. We finally had an admission date for the hospital. Now everything was hurry up. Six months since her diagnosis, but now everything had to be done in two weeks— harvest the bone marrow, fix her teeth, install a larger portacath.

We were at the surgeon's, the one who would install a new portacath, a bigger portacath. It was one-thirty, and we had a noon appointment.

"Sit down," the receptionist replied curtly. "He'll be with you shortly."

An hour later, we were rushed into his office.

"Sorry for the delay," he greeted us matter-of-factly. "Now let's . . ."

"Well, it's not all right," I replied politely, but firmly.

His face froze. His ears twitched as he tried to understand what he was hearing. "I had an emergency."

"Yes, yes. We all have emergencies," I responded. "But if someone is waiting for you, you call. That's only common courtesy."

"But I'm a doctor." His face took on a bewildered look. "I had an emergency," he repeated.

"And if your receptionist had told us you had an emergency, we could have gone out and had some lunch." It was now two-thirty and we had not eaten, as we had planned on having lunch after the appointment. Instead, we sat for two-and-a-half hours in a waiting room, trying to pry information from a receptionist who would only say that the doctor would see us shortly. It was not important to them whether we had eaten or not—they could not feel our hunger.

The doctor thought for a moment. "I suppose you could have eaten. I'm sorry."

He wasn't sincere.

"We could have kept our dentist appointment upstairs, too," I added. "Now we have to reschedule that and come back to Boston another day."

"I said I was sorry," he whined. "What more do you want?"

I wanted him to understand. I wanted him to tell his patients when he was running late. I wanted him to look at us as though we were human.

He botched the operation. I doubt he did it intentionally, but he botched it. A blood clot formed in my wife's arm, and her outpatient surgery became an ordeal. They rushed her back into surgery, informing me that she would have to stay overnight.

"You said it would be outpatient surgery," I complained to the doctor.

"Yes, but this is an emergency," he replied.

"You seem to have a lot of them."

His eyes had a vacant, confused look as he stared back at me. No, his failure hadn't been intentional. He didn't even remember the conversation we'd had earlier in his office.

While they had her in the hospital, they decided to pull four of her teeth. They didn't like the way they looked—sources of infection—and knowing her bone marrow would soon be gone, decided to pull them. There wasn't enough time to fix them properly, so they yanked them out instead. Six months of waiting, but there wasn't enough time to fix four teeth.

She was released from the hospital, but had to return to the blood center every day for two weeks and sit for four hours hooked up to a machine. The machine took her blood out through her new portacath and searched through it for bits of bone marrow—stem cells, they called them. It dripped the stem cells into a plastic bag, then put the rest of the blood back through her old portacath.

My bionic woman.

It was the last day of bone marrow harvesting, and they needed to do x–rays afterward. My instructions were to pick my wife up at the radiology waiting room.

I entered the waiting room and looked around. It was empty. The receptionist sat reading a magazine with a bride on the cover.

"Excuse me," I said. "I'm here for my wife."

She pushed her magazine down just enough for me to see her eyes. "She's not here."

"She has to be," I replied pleasantly. "She told me to meet her here."

"Well, look around," the receptionist said coldly. "There's nobody here."

I looked around. Eight plastic chairs and a print of a hibiscus mounted in a pink plastic frame, but no people. Certainly not my wife.

"Maybe they're still taking her x–rays?" I suggested.

"No." She moved her magazine back up so she wouldn't have to look at me. "There's no one back there."

Another woman walked up behind her, and the two huddled for a moment.

The other woman walked over to me. "They rolled her off on a gurney," she explained.

"To where?" I asked, incredulously.

The other woman looked over at the first woman. The magazine still covered her face. "To where?" she yelled.

"Emergency room, I think." The first woman lowered the magazine long enough to reply, then covered her face once more.

I dashed from the waiting area. What now? The hospital was a labyrinth of hallways, a collection of buildings connected without a plan by long, blind hallways, the walls painted yellow and lit with long rows of fluorescent lights. Yellow–tiled floors. So much yellow, you might think you were running down the insides of the fluorescent tubes themselves.

I found the emergency room, but they knew nothing about my wife.

"Try ambulatory care," someone yelled as I stood frozen in a whirl of activity.

I dashed back into the shimmering yellow tubes, frantic as I followed the signs to ambulatory care, casting sideways glances at the gurneys that lined the walls, scanning the faces of the sallow patients that slept upon them.

"Try the emergency room," someone in ambulatory care suggested.

This was not working.

I raced to the main lobby and leaned across the information desk, breathing heavily. "They've lost my wife!"

"Is she in–patient?" the volunteer asked.

"No, but I am," I replied angrily.

She looked at me funny. "In patient," she said.

"Oh, I thought you said . . . never mind," I shook my head. "No, she's out–patient."

"We only track those who are in–patient."

I stood back from the desk and stared up at the large map painted on the wall behind her, my vision blurred by the mixture of odd lighting and anger. Eighteen buildings, some twenty stories high. She was in there somewhere.

I leaned across the desk again. "Do you have any suggestions?"

"If she's not in–patient, then she's not in the computer."

"No, she's not in the computer," I said in exasperation, and turned toward the blood center, to where my wife had begun the day's journey.

"There you are!" It was an unfamiliar face that called to me, but I recognized the bride on the magazine that she still clutched. "I'm so sorry for the confusion. Your wife was in the x–ray room all along." She laughed, but I didn't laugh with her. "She came out just after you left, and I've been running around like a lunatic looking for you."

I returned to radiology and found my wife sitting calmly under the hibiscus print.

"I'm sorry I let the insurance company talk us into using this hospital," I greeted her. "It's a real zoo."

"You could have said no," she replied, gathering together a large collection of papers from the seat beside her.

"Well, they said if we came here, they'd pay for everything." The case worker had said that when he called. I informed him that the transplant doctor was not in their network, but he said that was okay—they had a good deal with the hospital, so if we went there, they'd pay for everything. He gave me an authorization number, advising me to keep it in case there was any question about payment.

I normally didn't write confirmation numbers down, but this time I did.

"Well, just two more days of this," I groaned as I helped her from her chair.

"Two more days of out–patient," she said. "Then I move in for the summer."

I held her hand gently as she gazed once more about the yard. A sadness filled her eyes as she looked down at the large green buds of the peonies, already beginning to droop under their weight.

"I hate doctors," she said. "They stalled all winter, and now I have to spend summer in the hospital." She touched one of the buds. "You'll remember to stake them?"

"The peonies?" I asked. "Of course."

She pulled away from me and knelt beside the pansies we had planted for quick color, nipped a dying bloom off between her fingernails and tossed it into the center of the lilies where it wouldn't be seen. "You'll pinch the dead flowers off everything, too? They'll bloom longer if you do that."

"Yes," I replied, and reached down for her hand once again. "We'd better get to the hospital."

As she took my hand, she looked up at the small gable of the third floor window and examined the tall ladder stretching up, touching the still-white shingles. "Perhaps you'll have the whole house painted by the time I get back," she said.

"I'll try," I promised.

She smiled sadly. "I make you work so hard. Don't I?"

"No."

"Always bossing you around."

"No. Just sharing thoughts," I said.

She stood up and threw her arms around my neck. "Don't go up on that ladder unless my mother's here," she cried. "I don't want anything happening to you."

Her mother couldn't catch me if I fell from that height, but I didn't say that. Instead, I whispered, "Don't worry about us." But I knew that she would.

She looked around once more and said good-bye to the approaching summer.

"You'll be home before you know it," I said. And summer will be waiting for you.

Chapter 18

❦

"SEE? OVER THERE." I stared southward as I stood in the window.

We were eight floors up, and in the distance we could see downtown. We could see the morning sun, a reflection in the mirrored façade of the downtown skyscrapers.

"The shiny black building to the left of the gold dome, that's my building."

She looked across the neighboring roofs. Laundry hung along the rooftops. Toward the hill, house plants and patio furniture sat on the flat roofs, occasionally framed in by glass boxcars that functioned as sun rooms for those who could afford them. Toward the sea were the high rises of the financial district.

"That little black sliver there?" She pointed to where I was looking.

I followed the angle of her arm and looked off the tip of her finger. "Yes. That's my building."

"Can I see your office from here?" she asked, her voice rising hopefully as though that would mean something.

"No. I'm on the other side of the building," I explained. "But the phone's right there. You can call me whenever you want."

"I don't want to be a bother," she sighed.

"You could never be a bother," I said.

I wanted to ask her whether or not she was scared, but a nurse hovered in the background, impatient to prepare my wife for her lethal infusion. Under normal circumstances it would kill the patient, but they were prepared: at the last moment, they would inject her with her own bone marrow and rescue her, bringing her back from the brink of death.

But what if they had lost her bone marrow? I wanted to see the bag of bone marrow they had spent the last two weeks collecting. I wanted to hold it and see her name typed professionally on a label and pasted firmly to the bag. I wanted to put the bag under a microscope and watch the bone marrow swim around. I wanted to see it swim around and know that it was still alive.

I was silent with my fears, though. They were just the irrational wanderings of an unsettled mind, like the traveler boarding an airplane worried that it might crash. But airplanes do crash.

Instead, I pointed to my office building as if we were tourists in the big city for the first time. "I'll stop in each morning before work just to say hi. Then I'll come and stay longer at lunch time. We can play cribbage or something."

Are you scared? I wanted to ask, but I didn't because there was no need to. Our thoughts were shared, locked together in a harmony that had brought us together in the first place, that held us together in a way that love was meant to be.

We were both scared.

"It's only a ten minute walk from my office, so if you ever want to see me, just call." I held her head between my finger-tips as I kissed her forehead, but all she felt was the paper surgical mask that covered my mouth. "You okay?"

She nodded her head uncertainly.

The nurse stared at me from a corner of the room, and told me with her fixed gray eyes that it was time to leave.

"I've got to get back to work." I opened the door to her room. It had a glass window, unusual for hospital doors. They were normally solid, but hers had a window so the nurses could look in without opening the door, without letting in germs and disease. It seemed like we were part of an experiment, as though space aliens wanted to learn how humans mated. They'd have to learn from someone else.

From the start, my wife wanted my blood, not a stranger's. She was worried; irony was a powerful force in the universe, and she was afraid that she would be cured of cancer only to come down with hepatitis or something even worse.

She told the doctors that she wanted my blood, but nobody told me I had to give it ahead of time. I visualized myself lying beside her on a matching cot as they poured my blood into hers through a connecting hose. "Leave a little for me," I'd joke—a dashing, heroic figure lying gallantly beside my wife.

"That's not how we do it," a nurse explained. It was two days after the lethal dose, and my wife's blood counts were seriously low. "It has to be processed and typed and labeled," she said as she hung a bag of stranger's blood on my wife's IV stand. "That all takes time."

My wife lay silent, barely conscious, unable to object. I stared at my eager veins bulging with anticipation, then reluctantly rolled my sleeve back down.

"She'll need your platelets more than anything," the nurse whispered as we tiptoed around the ashen-faced patient. "I'll call and get you an appointment."

My wife did not stir. I stared down at her, thinking she looked dead.

The nurse saw my concern. "She's doing really well," she informed me, her voice professional yet sympathetic.

I stared at her lying there, unmoving, and wondered what she would have looked like if she were doing poorly. I wondered, too, what she had been like the day before. My wife requested that I not visit her then, and I honored her wish. But the nurse said she was doing really well, which implied some sort of improvement. I shuddered as I thought how close to death she must have come.

There was a wastepaper basket outside my wife's door. Each time I left, I removed the paper hat from my head, the paper booties from my shoes, and the surgical mask from my face, crumpled them up into a big blue ball, and tossed them into the basket. That was her protection against the outside world— paper booties, paper masks, paper hats. Anyone wanting to enter her room had to suit up first.

Above the basket was a sink with liquid soap and detailed washing instructions in bold print taped to a mirror. Those who didn't care to wash could put on latex gloves.

The nurses always used the gloves.

"That's because they come in here all the time," my wife explained to me when I returned on Sunday. "Their skin would crack if they washed that much."

She was talking again. She didn't want to talk about her recent medical experience—her brush with death—so we talked about soap.

"You mean they'd have to wash every time?" I asked.

"Every time," she replied. She moved her peg to the end of the cribbage board. "I didn't skunk you this time," she remarked as she slid the board away.

"You don't want to play another one?" I asked.

"No." She closed her eyes and lay her head back against her pillow.

"You're tired," I whispered. "I'll let you sleep."

She didn't respond.

I stood up and walked slowly to the door. Safely outside, my germs successfully corralled and stuffed into the wastepaper basket, I looked back through the window and stared at my wife lying there breathing quietly.

She's getting better, I told myself, and turned away to return home to our daughter.

Chapter 19

*S*HE HEARD ME COME IN, recognizing my
footsteps with as much certainty as if I had spoken, and her
eyes flitted opened. Her hand slid along the rail of her bed,
feeling for the controls.

"I wish we had one of these at home," she said as she
pushed a button.

I heard the whirl of a motor, and the head end of her bed
began to rise.

Without thinking, I reached out to stroke her hair, then
pulled back, fearful that germs might linger under my fingernails. Instead I blew her a kiss.

"They posted my blood chart today." She pointed to a spot
on the wall just below the television set. "That means I'm out
of the woods."

I looked to where she was pointing and saw the white sheet of paper stuck to the wall with two thumb tacks. A length of yarn dangled from one thumb tack, and a yellow pencil was tied to the end.

"That's what that means?" I said.

"Sure," she replied. "They don't put it up until you're out of the woods because they don't want you seeing your blood counts collapse."

The door opened, and a kitchen aide brought in a lunch tray.

"The food here is pretty good for a hospital," my wife remarked, lifting the tin dish cover and examining the contents. "I guess this is what I ordered."

She sipped happily at her pasteurized juice as I shuffled the deck of cards. "The nurse should be in soon with today's blood counts."

The door opened again. It was the kitchen aide returning with the salt she had forgotten the first time.

Salt isn't good for you, I was going to say, but realized how foolish that would sound to a woman who had just had a lethal dose of chemo drugs surging through her veins.

I dealt out a hand of cribbage, but our eyes kept straying from the cards to the door, seeking the nurse with the blood counts.

The door opened again. We both watched as a woman in white entered, hoping she would head toward the chart. Instead, she went to the toilet and poured urine from the bed pan into a measuring cup.

"Looks like those kidneys are functioning all right," the nurse laughed, then blushed slightly when she realized she was in mixed company.

"Here we are." Another nurse had snuck in as we watched the first one pour urine. This new nurse was cheerful yet businesslike as she marched up to the blood chart and began writing on it. "Looking good. Looking good."

I set my cards down and drifted over to see what she was doing.

"Oh!" the nurse shouted, startled to find me standing so near. "You're the husband?"

I nodded my head.

"Well, these are your wife's blood counts. Each day we draw some blood so we can measure her white blood cells, red blood cells, and platelets." She poked the chart with her pencil each time she mentioned a type of blood. "Then we mark them here on this graph." She looked at the chart with a certain amount of pleasure. "Your wife is looking pretty good."

I looked at the chart. "They're going down, though." Perhaps they had hung the chart upside down. No, upside down would still show them going down. Perhaps they had hung it sideways. I tipped my head to one side—that was better.

"They will drop at first, until her bone marrow grows back." The nurse traced lightly along the dots with her pencil. "They've leveled off, though. See?"

I nodded my head.

"What's the red mark?" I asked.

"When all her counts are above that red line, she can go home," the nurse explained. "If you have proper support at home." She stared at me, wondering whether a man was capable of giving proper support.

"Her mother has moved in with us," I replied, and the nurse relaxed. Ah yes, a woman—there was proper support.

I studied the chart too long for the little information it held. It was a long way from the three new pencil marks at the bottom of the chart to the red line near the top.

"Once they start giving you my blood, those lines will shoot straight up." I smiled at my wife and rejoined her in my chair beside her bed.

The cribbage game no longer interested us, and I put the cards away.

"I'm giving platelets this afternoon," I mentioned as she sipped the last of her pasteurized juice. I had been suffering an uneasy feeling, that I had let my wife down, ever since the blood incident. All she had wanted was my blood, yet now strangers were keeping her alive. I was hoping that once in the blood center, as the nurses relieved me of my platelets, they would also relieve me of my guilt.

"You better go then," she said. "You don't want to be away from the office for too long." She pulled the pegs from the cribbage board—the game barely started, interrupted by our desire to watch the progress of her chart.

I stood up, leaned over her bed, and kissed her through the paper mask. It was not enough. I wanted to lift the mask from my mouth and feel her soft cheek against my lips.

Alone in the crowd of the hospital's main floor—a shuffling mass of faceless people—I wandered through the yellow halls. Approaching from the distance was her current doctor, the head of bone marrow transplants.

"Hello, doctor," I said.

His pencil-thin mustache twitched once. His stethoscope bounced out from his stomach as though it recognized me, but he looked straight through me and kept on walking, dragged along by a hungry mob headed for the cafeteria.

I followed the signs directing the way to the blood center, detouring around the ever-present construction projects, feeling that I was going in a circle, that I would be stuck looping around and around forever. In the distance, though, the light changed, and I found myself in the sterile lobby of the blood center.

I was led to an alcove where a pleasant nurse hooked me up to the pheresis machine, the same one they had used to harvest my wife's bone marrow. The same nurse who had siphoned my wife siphoned me. It gave me a peculiar sense of closeness to my wife.

The nurse pushed a needle into my right arm and strapped it to my skin with surgical tape so it wouldn't move. She stabbed a sharp plastic tube into my left arm. The needle was relatively painless, but the tube hurt. She taped the plastic tube to my left arm and stabilized it. Even then it hurt, but I thought of my wife, and I thought of her pain. It didn't make my pain feel any less, but it did make me feel like more of a sissy.

"Here's some Tums," the nurse said.

I took them, held them in my hand, stared at them. "What are these for?"

"Calcium loss," she explained. "The process depletes your calcium, and your face might tingle. The Tums help."

It sounded a bit foolish. I set the Tums on the little table beside me, then watched, intrigued, as the blood flowed from my right arm, through the clear plastic tube. I couldn't see it as it traveled behind me through the coils of tubing, fluttering about in the strange centrifugal machine until the machine had taken what it wanted. But I picked the route up again as the bright red liquid traveled back to my left arm and back into my body where it belonged.

The nurse left for a few minutes. My face started feeling funny. Not ha-ha funny, but tingly funny. Nurse, nurse! I reached for the Tums, but it was too late. I quickly grabbed the arms of my chair for support instead.

Earthquake.

It was like I was sitting on top of a washing machine. Nurse, nurse! I wanted to yell, but my mouth wouldn't work. Where was that nurse? What was happening to the building? I felt like I was riding a train, strapped to the front of the locomotive. My lips quivered, my cheeks shook, my eyes vibrated.

The nurse walked in.

"Tu-u-u-u-u-u-u-ums," I groaned.

"Are you tingling?" she asked as she plucked one of the Tums from the little table.

"Ye-e-e-e-e-s." I opened my mouth, the nurse placed the Tums on my tongue, and the shaking gradually subsided. "That was wild."

"Oh? Did you feel a tingle?" she asked as she checked the level of platelets in the collection bag. "Next time, have milk or something before you come. For the calcium."

I entered her room and went instinctively to the blood chart before kissing her. "Your counts are inching up."

"Did you give platelets yesterday?" she asked.

I rolled up my sleeves and showed her the Band-Aids on my arms.

"You can't take them off yet?" she asked.

"I'm leaking," I replied. "I gave you all my platelets, so now I'm leaking."

"What a martyr," she laughed. "You brought me magazines?"

I showed her the stack. "I didn't read them. They're fresh— no germs," I said. I sat down in a chair beside the window and stared at her, afraid to touch her even after washing my hands, afraid I'd convey to her some wretched subway germ.

"How's everything at home?" she asked.

"Fine," I said. "Your mother cooked dinner. Something with shrimp in it."

"And peas?" she asked.

I nodded.

"Shrimp wiggle. One of her specialties." She smiled at me. "But you don't eat shrimp. Did you eat any?"

"A little," I said. "I pretended they were crunchy mushrooms."

"Wait until she makes you woodcock," she warned. "It looks like vomit."

124

"She means well," I replied, then gazed longingly at my wife's face. "I miss you."

Her hair was falling out again, and she wanted me to chop it off.

"It just fell out from the Taxol," I said. I snipped at her short reddish hair with dull scissors as her mashed potatoes grew cold on the rolling table beside her bed.

"It's falling out again," she replied. She had moved from the bed to an armchair and was sitting up. When she got tired of that spot, she would move from the armchair back to the bed. Later, she would move to the armchair again.

The armchair was a good place for haircuts.

"Yeah, but it just grew back," I remarked as I continued snipping.

"But it's falling back out."

"I don't understand," I whined. "Why does cancer build up immunity to this stuff but hair doesn't?"

"Because it's cancer," she replied, "not hair."

Secretly, I was pleased that her hair was falling out again. It was a sign that something was happening inside her. The drugs were out and about—seek and destroy—and cancer was dying along with the hair.

"Won't the hospital staff cut your hair?" I asked.

"They would," she sighed contentedly. "But I'd rather have you do it."

The kitchen aide entered the room and picked up my wife's lunch tray.

"Hey," I snapped. "She's not done."

The aide looked at her watch. "Twenty minutes is up." Then she took the tray away.

"What is this? A prison camp?" I asked angrily.

"They only give me twenty minutes to eat," my wife explained. "Bacteria starts forming on the food after that."

I was going to keep that in mind when I had supper. I didn't want to eat bacteria either. Shrimp wiggle was hard enough to eat.

"Done." I stood back and looked at her hair. It had that chopped look I'd seen in an old World War II movie, where the women were sheared by the partisans because they had slept with the enemy. "Now you look more like a prisoner of war."

"I usually wear a bandanna anyway," she said. She looked at the results in a hand mirror. "Keep your day job."

I stuck my tongue out at her, and that made her laugh. "They're expecting me at the blood center," I said. "I'd better go."

"Again?" she asked. "How often can you give?"

"You can give platelets every forty-eight hours."

"I'll be able to see right through you soon," she said as she followed me to the door.

From the hallway, I threw her a kiss. She pressed her fingers up against the glass, and I pressed mine to meet hers, separated by an invisible force field.

I love you, she mouthed.

My lips moved in reply. I love you the most.

I love you like toast.

Chapter 20

*S*HE ATE HER LUNCH FIRST, before we did anything else. I timed the kitchen aide—twenty-two minutes. She was late. I studied the peas that my wife left behind, swimming in butter sauce, and wondered if any bacteria had formed yet.

"How are things at home?" she asked after placing the tin cover over her plate, a signal to the aide that she was done. It was Thursday, day six in transplant lingo. Six days since her bone marrow had been re-introduced into her body.

"Four-year-olds are a bit strange," I observed as I dealt each of us seven cards, then set the remainder of the deck on the rolling table.

"Oh?" She arranged her cards, then pulled one from the top of the deck.

"She won't go near your mother," I said. "She thinks she's there to replace you."

She threw a seven-of-clubs on the discard pile, and I snatched it up.

"Collecting sevens, are we?" she asked softly, almost to herself as if to mark that fact in her mind. She thought of what I had said. "Well, she is there to replace me, isn't she?"

"Not permanently, though," I said.

"We'll see."

There had been an odd coolness from our daughter toward her grandmother. It was a coolness that told me that our daughter understood more of what was going on than we had believed.

"Grammy is coming to visit for a while," I explained.

I had said it enthusiastically, but the little girl did not respond. She continued coloring fish in a Sea World coloring book as she sat on the living room floor, the television set blaring in front of her.

Too many distractions, I thought, and turned the television off with the remote. "Did you hear me?" I asked. "Grammy's coming."

"Uh huh." She didn't look up, but scribbled harder until the crayon broke.

I shrugged.

When I was a boy, a visit from my grandmother was an exciting event. She was ancient. She had lived in another era—a mysterious era—and she had outgrown her desire to punish children, mellowing with age like a fine antique.

"No use crying over spilt milk," my grandma would say calmly, while my mother dabbed a washcloth at my shirt sleeve, clutching it with her angry fingers, asking whether I thought she liked spending all her time doing laundry.

She'll cheer up once she sees her grandmother, I thought. When the time arrived, though, she stayed up in her room.

"Grammy's here!" I called, but there was silence from the floor above. "Get down here!" I yelled angrily, then flashed a pleasant smile at my mother-in-law. "She's been talking about you all morning."

"Hi, dear." My mother-in-law kissed my cheek, then patted my shoulder, but said nothing more as I set her luggage next to the stairs and led her into the living room.

The little girl waged her silent battle, her grandmother an innocent target. She came downstairs, marched past her grandmother, and kissed me as the two of us sat together on the sofa. Then she turned around and marched past her again, to the other end of the room, and picked up her dolls one at a time, glancing back over her shoulder to be sure that we noticed as she kissed each one of them.

"She does love you," I reassure my mother-in-law.

"Of course she does," she replied. "It's hard on her, though, with all that's going on."

"Your mother will be home soon," I yelled toward my daughter. "She's going to get better, and she's going to watch you grow up into a teenager, and the two of you are going to have horrific fights."

The little girl stared at me briefly, then kissed another doll. "Come, Bobo."

"No," I said. "Bobo can't play with you until you're nice to your grammy."

The little girl started to cry.

"It's all right," my mother-in-law said. "I understand."

But could she understand? A four-year-old certainly couldn't understand. I couldn't understand. Could anyone understand?

I thought the two would bond in time, but they didn't.

"You shrank my favorite shirt!" the little girl cried, halfway between anger and a sob.

"No, I think it's okay." Her grandmother tried to put it on her, but the little girl wouldn't get near enough for her to button it up. "You'll have to move closer, dear."

The washing machine buzzed, calling my mother-in-law into the basement.

"Why are you so mean to your grammy?" I asked, once my daughter and I were alone.

"I don't know," she replied, her voice quivering.

"You should be glad she's visiting," I said. "She can teach you how to bake cookies."

"She can't cook." Tears were forming in her eyes.

"Who says your grammy can't cook?"

"Mommy does." The mention of her mother opened the floodgates. She could no longer hold back the tears. She ran into my arms and cried silently.

"She cried because my mother can't cook?" My wife was no longer looking at her cards, but was staring at me as I told her the story.

"I think she needs to see you," I said. "Do you feel well enough to see her tomorrow?"

"What's tomorrow?" she asked as she picked up my discard and stuck it between her last two cards.

"Saturday," I answered, drawing another card from the top of the deck.

She looked at me like I had said something stupid.

"Day eight, I think," I said, converting to a calendar that had more meaning to my wife.

"Bring her. It should be safe." She pulled a final card from the deck, then smiled at me. "Gin."

I swept the cards from the table and stuffed them back into

their box. "I've got to go," I remarked briskly. "Platelets again."

This time I lowered the paper mask and kissed her cheek, the first time our skin had met in more than a week. It felt cold—she needed my warm blood.

Downstairs I had a different nurse—a man—but my regular nurse stood nearby, watching us discreetly as she worked on another donor.

"You here again?" she asked as the unfamiliar male fingers tapped at my arm, investigating my veins. Sewer pipes, the nurses called them. We love your arms—your veins are like sewer pipes!

"They said out front I can donate platelets every forty-eight hours," I replied casually.

"Well, what they say and what we say are two different things," the woman nurse huffed. "And what we say is what counts."

The male nurse went about his task with expert precision, punching needles into my arms, threading the plastic hose, calibrating. He did not concern himself with whether or not I should be there—he would let the machine decide that.

"Tums," I said, and pointed to the Paul Bunyan-size jug sitting on a shelf below the television set.

"You want the TV on?" he asked, noticing the vacant set as he grabbed the Tums. He didn't wait for my answer, but turned it on out of habit, then lay the small speaker on the pillow beside my head as he placed a fistful of Tums into my hand. "Enough?"

It was an older television, with no remote control and apparently only one channel. The last session, I watched two hours of weather and learned the temperature in Bangkok. Ninety-eight degrees. (It's not the heat, though. It's the humidity.)

"If you've been hurt in an accident," I heard a man's voice

saying as I turned up the volume, "you are entitled to compensation." An advertisement. A lawyer out trolling for sprained ankles and stiff necks. Babies. Sissies. Ask my wife about pain and suffering. Ask her if there's anything that would compensate for her pain.

"Turn it off, please" I called.

The nurse shrugged, then walked over and flicked it off.

I put on a set of headphones and dialed around for suitable music—bloodletting music, something soothing, but not too sad. Closing my eyes, I thought of far-away places, dreamed of Montana where we honeymooned at Glacier National Park. I dreamed of the peacefulness of Thomson Meadow and how my wife worried about grizzlies after stepping on a bear poop.

"But I have this grizzly stick," I told her, and shook it so the little bell tied to the handle rang out.

"How's that going to stop a bear?" she asked.

"They hear the bell ringing, and they run away," I explained.

I felt the hot breath of a grizzly, but opened my eyes and saw it was the nurse taking the needle from my arm.

"Got all you need already?" I asked.

"No," he said. "Your platelets are too low. See?" He showed me a computer printout that I did not understand. The machine had made its decision.

"But my wife needs my platelets," I cried.

"You can't do this all by yourself." The woman nurse had entered the little alcove and was helping the male nurse unstrap my arms. "You must have family or friends who can donate," she suggested.

Ten minutes later, she found me sitting in one of the big, brown vinyl chairs in the large, sunny room where they drew blood.

"Now what are you doing?" she asked impatiently.

"I'm giving blood," I replied. "I haven't given whole blood

for six weeks. They said out front that I could still give whole blood."

"Go home," she ordered. "You can't do this all by yourself."

I called my wife from my office and told her what had happened, that I had failed. She would be getting stranger's blood again soon.

"Call my sisters. They want to donate," she replied. "I'd call them myself, but it would be too weird asking someone for blood."

"It would be weird for me to ask for blood, too," I said.

"No, that's different," she argued. "You'd be asking for blood for someone else."

It was weird, though. I called one of her sisters and asked for some of her blood.

"When do you want us? Tonight?"

"As soon as possible," I replied.

"Then tonight," she said. "We've been waiting for your call. I'll phone the others and we'll all drive in together after dinner."

I saw then that they were anxious to help, grateful to be given a role in their sister's battle. It was not weird to need their blood.

Swiftly, they put their plan into action, all meeting at the designated house at the proper time as though it were a maneuver they had practiced time and again. One adult—an incompatible blood type—stayed behind to watch the children while the others marched off toward the city.

Blood was spilled that night, but it was for a noble cause.

Chapter 21

*T*HE SOUNDS OUTSIDE my bedroom window were those of morning. Not the dark silence that usually greeted me when I slipped outside with my paint brush, but birds singing and children giggling, sweetened by the morning sun. I had overslept.

My mother-in-law fixed my daughter her breakfast while I stayed in bed listening. Words, sounds of the older female voice drifted up to my room. The little-girl voice was silent. From what I could hear, I knew that my daughter was refusing to eat.

Coming down the stairs, tugging at the pajamas worn for my mother-in-law's benefit, wishing for the baggy underpants that were my preferred Saturday morning garb, I walked into the kitchen and touched my daughter's head.

"Hi, Dada," she said.

"You're alone," I remarked, looking about and seeing that my mother-in-law had left the kitchen.

"No. Elizabeth, Sally, and Patty are here," she replied, referring to her invisible sisters. Patty was almost eight. Bobo was out back with an invisible bone.

"Eat," I said. "We're going to see your mother in a little while." I looked around, rubbing the sleep from my eyes, and heard the familiar sound of the washing machine filling with water in the basement. My mother-in-law was doing laundry again.

"You make my breakfast."

"Eat." I pointed at her plate, the bagel and cream cheese, the grapefruit with each section carefully sliced from the rind.

"Make me something else," she replied.

I shook my head as I poured water into a coffee cup and set it in the microwave. "You can wear your pretty dress and your pretty shoes," I said. "But your stomach will growl if you don't eat. That's not pretty."

"No it won't." She laughed.

"It will. Now eat." I had to use my daddy voice.

"Make my breakfast for me?" she pleaded. "Please." There were tears behind her voice now.

I picked up her bagel, scraped the cream cheese off with my finger, then spread new cream cheese on with the knife her grandmother had used. I waited for her to complain about the used knife, but she didn't. "Here. Now eat so your stomach doesn't growl."

A pretty dress was usually enough to get her going, but the hospital was something scary. She had not been to one since her birth, but she knew that the hospital was a scary place. It took more than a fancy dress and shiny black shoes to make her a willing visitor.

≫≪

"Daddy's going to buy me a balloon afterward." She sat carefully in a corner chair with her knees pulled up to her chest, her dress pulled out and over her knees so that only her ankles showed. She had been unhappy about wearing a mask at first, but now she liked it—it reminded her of trick-or-treating. The mask was a bit large for a child, though, and kept sliding about her face as she talked.

Her mother lay on her bed toward the middle of the room, almost sitting, propped up by pillows, the blanket and sheet pulled up only as far as her waist. A television hovered over her with the sound turned off, blue images flashing from the picture tube, just enough to distract me and draw my eyes toward the ceiling as we spoke.

"They didn't do your blood test yet?" I asked.

"They did," she replied. "But they haven't come back with the results yet."

My wife's sisters had been in the night before and tried to decorate the room for our daughter's visit. Pink curtains hung in the window, and several vases of flowers sat on the window sill, daffodils drooping from the heat of the morning sun. I looked toward the window and tried to pretend we were in a cheap motel, not a hospital room, but the periodic crackle of the hospital intercom prevented the illusion from taking hold.

"Come give your mommy a hug," my wife pleaded. She held out her arms and tried to look inviting, but the little girl was too scared.

Instead, our daughter stared at the two IV stands that stood beside the hospital bed. "Maybe Daddy will buy me two balloons afterward," she said cautiously, and pulled her knees tighter to her chest.

"You little operator," my wife laughed. "Come here and give your mommy a hug."

The barrier cracked from the gentle laughter, and the little girl ran to the bed, quickly, hoping to get there before fear could overtake her. She leaned over and hugged her mother, and before she knew what had happened, my wife scooped her into the bed with her. They lay there, my wife smiling at her child as she held the little head tight against her breast, our daughter rigid, with unblinking eyes.

"Oh, go on! Get out of here," my wife shouted happily. "It's too nice of a day to hang out in a hospital room."

The little girl rolled off the bed and ran toward the door without a complaint. "Come on, Daddy. Mommy says it's all right to go now."

"In a minute." I needed to wait for the nurse to come in and mark the chart, to show where the blood counts were now. Every day they had been inching up closer and closer to the red line, a map tracing the progress of my prisoner wife as she tunneled toward freedom.

"Come on, Daddy!"

The nurse entered and glided silently across the room to the chart. "Let's see." Ever so slowly, she placed the three marks on the chart, then continued standing in front of it as she connected the prior day's dots to the new ones, blocking my view with her wide shoulders.

I came up behind her quietly and stared over her right shoulder. "Ninety on the platelets," I said. "Looking good."

The nurse jumped a bit, once again startled that someone was so close to her, then turned and smiled briefly at me. "Looks great," she agreed. "Keep it up, and you can go home in a week or so." She looked at me. "If there's proper support at home."

"My mother's living with us for now," my wife explained.

A second nurse entered the room and hung two more bags from one of the IV stands; one was filled with a rich red liquid, the other with a creamy yellow fluid. I wondered if the yellow fluid was my platelets, whether they had finally processed, typed, and labeled mine and brought it up here for my wife.

Our daughter stared briefly at the bags of fluid, a look of distrust showing in her sideways glance. "Come on, Daddy. You said you'd buy me a balloon," she whined as she rattled the door knob, threatening to leave on her own.

I turned from the chart. Three little dots—all the information we would get on a daily basis. I always stared too long at them, looking for answers they couldn't provide.

I walked to my wife and kissed her. "I'll see you tomorrow."

"Come alone, though." She pointed toward our daughter. "The hospital frightens her."

I nodded my head, then strode to our daughter and lifted her up onto my shoulders. "Tomorrow at noon," I said to my wife, then carried the little girl from the room, ducking as we went together through the open door. "You get three balloons, Pumpkin," I promised as I shut the door behind us.

Outside the door, we turned once more toward my wife. We both waved through the doorway window at her as she lay there in the hospital bed, the two nurses moving about, adjusting IV tubes and measuring urine.

My daughter said, "I love you, Mommy," too softly for my wife to hear through the thick glass of the window. But she read the child's lips and smiled.

We held hands as we walked, my daughter's sure footsteps leading me toward the elevator.

"Don't you want to come see your mommy again?"

"Nope," she replied. "She'll be home soon."

"It may be a while," I warned.

"She'll be home soon," she said confidently, and began swinging our hands in a wide arc, like a smile.

Chapter 22

W E MARKED THE REMAINDER of her stay
with morning newspapers, twenty-minute lunches, and a seem-
ingly endless string of cribbage and gin rummy. And always
looking at the chart, watching the blood counts climb toward
the red line—the red line that would set her free.

Finally, the door burst open with an odd ring to it, as if
heralding an announcement, and we both set our cards down
to look at the bold figure standing in the doorway.

"You can go home tomorrow," the nurse's voice rang out as
she stepped into the room and sauntered to the chart to place
dots above the red line with exaggerated motions of her pencil. "The social worker will review everything with you at nine.
Then we'll have a little party."

"Then I can go home?" she begged. She wasn't ungrateful—a party was nice—but she just wanted to go home.

The nurse turned to face us, smiled, and nodded her head eagerly.

They opened the door to her room once more. It opened just as it had opened a hundred times before, but this time it was followed by a whoosh, like the vacuum in a coffee can. It was freedom flooding the room.

Whoosh, my butterfly, you're free!

One of the nurses had made pink frosted cupcakes, but my wife wouldn't eat any.

"I'm too nervous to eat." She stared at the tray of cupcakes but left her protective surgical mask in place.

A woman shook her hand while two others patted her back, their latex gloves a gentle reminder that my wife was not entirely free, that she was merely leaving one protective cocoon to enter another. But the other was at least her own home where she would be among her family once again.

Together we headed toward the elevator, just as my daughter and I had walked hand-in-hand two weekends before.

I looked across at the wig that hid her bald head, and watched as she cautiously moved her feet across the glittering tile floor, as if entering a forbidden land. Her eyes darted about, looking up at the corners of the hallway, searching for germs missed by the orderlies in their daily cleaning.

The elevator door opened—it was empty—and we stepped in.

"I'm going home," she said softly. "Finally."

"Only eighteen days." I pressed the button to the lobby. "That was pretty good."

"Eighteen days was a long time," she remarked.

"But at least it wasn't a month."

Her recovery had been without incident, except for a minor bout with fluid in her lungs. They called it pneumonia, but she was so full of antibiotics that it never stood a chance.

"It looks nice," she said as we pulled into the driveway. It was not just being home that she commented on. I had been painting the house while she was away.

One hour each morning. One hour, then off to work. It didn't seem like enough time to accomplish much, but slowly the ladders worked their way around the first corner of the house. By the time my wife came home from the hospital, the ladders stood at the far end of the second side, casting their shadows across the parlor's bay window. If we stood together in just the right spot and placed our cheeks against each other's, there was the illusion that the entire house had been painted, that the job was done and mornings could be spent in bed again.

"You like it?" I held her elbow as we approached the porch steps.

"It looks lovely." She hurried up the stairs onto the side porch, happy to be home after eighteen days in the hospital.

I held the door open. "I guess we have to start counting again."

"The first hundred days," she said. "Eighty two to go."

"No. Not the hundred days. The two years."

A hundred days was how long she had to stay inside, restricting her activities, isolating herself the best she could from the outside world.

I followed her and watched as she roamed through the house, adjusting the dress on her Flapper Barbie Doll, picking up her grandmother's antique vase and feeling the smoothness of the glass. She stopped before the photograph of the two of us, taken just before our wedding—our engagement picture. "I've changed," she said.

"We've both changed," I replied. "But you've kept your beauty."

She pulled off her wig and laughed. "Oh yeah, a real beauty."

"That's just hair," I replied earnestly. "It hardly counts."

She reached the parlor. The emptiness reminded her of her hospital room, and she sat heavy in the inexpensive chair we had ordered through the JC Penny catalog. A rope swung gently against the window, hanging from the ladder outside.

"You're sad?" I asked as a placed a hand on her shoulder.

She nodded her head. "I shouldn't be. I'm home."

Home, but not safe, I thought. Had she dragged the danger home with her? Had one lone cancer cell sought refuge somewhere deep in her body where the drugs could not reach it? Only time would tell.

In one hundred days she could reenter the world. In two years she'd know if she was going to stay there.

"What are the chances that they killed every cell?" she asked nervously.

"They did," I assured her. "You'll live to be a hundred."

"They could be in me right now, growing somewhere," she remarked, staring nervously at her hands.

"They could be in me, too," I replied.

"Don't even think it." She rose from her seat and walked to her house plants. "You know, the odds are only twenty percent that I'm cured."

"Yes, but the odds of you getting breast cancer were only ten percent," I explained. "You're twice as likely to get cured as you were of get sick in the first place."

She shook her head. "I can't argue math," she replied. "Girls are never good at math." She was about to stick her finger in the soil to test for moisture, but she caught herself. Soil had germs. "Have you been watering my plants?"

"Every day," I said.

"That's too much," she scolded. "They'll drown."

We heard a car door outside and knew that our daughter had returned from her cousins' house where they had been playing under the sprinkler. We stood in the parlor and waited. My wife removed her wig again and dropped it on the JC Penny catalog chair.

"Aren't I beautiful?" she asked, rubbing her bald head as our daughter walked cautiously into the room still wearing her pink bathing suit.

The little girl stared for a moment, unsure, then threw her arms open and ran to my wife, her smile beaming to us her thoughts. Yes, Mommy, you're beautiful.

My wife came out onto the side porch—the limit of her world— and sat in a rocker. She watched us play, glancing over at her gardens, wanting to walk out among the flowers, to pull a few weeds just to feel a part of them once again. But the hundred days weren't up yet, and soil contained a huge assortment of unseen organisms.

"Can we go for a ride?" she asked. "I won't get out of the car."

"After our game," I promised as I tossed a Nerf ball toward the yellow Frisbee that served as home plate.

"Will you play nine innings?" she asked.

"Well, we're playing four strikes and you're out, two outs to an inning, so the rules are a little loose." I looked toward home plate, at our daughter. "Can we take Mommy for a ride?"

"Just one more hit," my daughter begged.

We drove along the coastal highway, hugging the jagged Maine shoreline wherever we could, viewing the sailboats and the white caps as they raced across the unnamed bays and coves. There was an old Civil War-era fort, abandoned before the war ended, before the fort was even finished, the rocks lying scattered about the field where the workmen had left them.

"There's no one here." She opened the car door and stepped gently to the ground. "Can we get out and walk around?"

She walked carefully among the grass and sat on a slab of stone looking out toward the scattered islands and the open sea.

I looked toward the parking lot, waiting for an encroaching vehicle to invade our solitude, prepared to grab my wife's arm and whisk her back to the hermetically-sealed safety of our van.

"It's too bad we live on the east coast," she sighed. "I'd like to see the sun set on the ocean."

"We'll go to the Cape someday," I replied. "We'll go to Wellfleet and watch the sun set there."

"Now?" she pleaded. "Let's go now."

"No," I said softly. "September."

That would have to wait until the fall, until after the hundredth day. Today you must work to get better, to live a hundred years, not a hundred days.

"We'll go in September," I promised.

I divided the medical bills into two piles—those that the insurance company paid correctly and those they had not. The ones they paid I filed away; the other ones I stuffed into my briefcase to bring to work. My employer was owned by my insurance carrier; any payment problems were work-related and would be dealt with on company time using company phones.

"What did they pay wrong?" my wife asked.

"Oh, all sorts of things," I replied. "They didn't pay the non-network doctor everything. Something about reasonable and customary."

"They do that so you don't go to some overpriced Holly-wood doctor," she explained.

"Yes, but they were the ones who chose that doctor." I leafed through the pile. "They didn't pay the blood tests because they went to an out-of-network lab."

"But those tests were done at the doctor's office," she said. "They have a machine right there."

"Apparently your doctor is in the network, but his equipment isn't," I replied. "Let's see. X-rays weren't covered because they were done out-of-network." I picked up our benefits booklet and leafed quickly through it. Yes, it was right there on page M-28: x-rays would be covered at network levels if there were no network facilities in the area. There were no network facilities in Boston. They would have to pay that one, too.

"What else didn't they pay?" she asked.

"Some clerical errors. They paid this doctor the first time, but they didn't pay the second time because they listed it as an outpatient service."

I thumbed through the correction pile and divided it into two piles as I went; the ones that would be easy to fix, and what I called the battlegrounds—the ones that I would have to learn all the rules. "They spelled this doctor's name wrong and couldn't find him in the computer." I put that one in the easy pile.

"I don't even remember him," she remarked. "But then

there were so many doctors coming in and out of my hospital room."

A nurse, a daily visitor, trotted about the kitchen as we talked. "Don't let those insurance companies push you around," she advised.

There was a red plastic bucket in the kitchen filled with discarded needles and pasted with a label warning of dangerous blood products inside. My wife's blood was not dangerous, unless something had happened in the hospital that they weren't telling us about. The bucket had a tight-fitting lid with a covered slot in it so the needles could be pushed in but they wouldn't come back out. The nurse shoved another needle through the slot. "Stick to your guns," she said. She had no specific advice, but was merely offering her moral support.

The two stacks of medical bills grew and shrank on my desk at work, depending on the cooperation of the insurance company.

"I have no control over where the doctor sends the blood," I shouted as my grip tightened around the telephone receiver.

"According to your policy, it's your responsibility to see that all tests go to network facilities," the clerk instructed.

"Gee, I was talking to the Attorney General this morning, and Bob said that setting conditions in a contract that one party couldn't be reasonably expected to fulfill would constitute fraud." I didn't know any Bobs, at least not any with a legal background.

"Let me ask my supervisor." Her voice was replaced by an accordion playing a familiar Beatle tune.

I looked down and saw my fingers drumming along on my desk to the beat of the accordion. Before I could tell my fingers to stop their ridiculous behavior, the sound of the accordion faded out and the clerk was back on the phone. "That was a mistake. It should have been paid." She paused for a brief second. "Thank you for calling."

"Wait! I've got more," I shouted.

The next one was the x-ray bill. I thought that would be a problem, but she said they had issued a memo just that morning addressing that problem—x-rays in Boston were to be paid at network levels.

"Any more?" she asked impatiently.

I read her the next service date and the provider, but I didn't understand the problem.

"That wasn't paid because that's a female procedure and you're a man," she explained.

"That's a mistake," I replied. "It should have listed my wife as the patient." A clerk had entered the policy holder as the patient. She could fix that one easily.

"Now, I've got this doctor charge, service date. . . ."

I heard her type it into the computer. A brief silence followed as she stared at her terminal and absorbed the information. "We don't pay above reasonable and customary," she explained.

"But your caseworker said if we went to this particular hospital and this particular doctor, you would pay all the charges," I replied.

"All the charges except above reasonable and customary."

"The caseworker didn't say that. He said 'all the charges.' I've got a reference number." I leafed quickly through my little notebook and found the number that had been read to me six months earlier.

"But we won't pay above reasonable and customary," she repeated. "Send us a letter if you wish to appeal," she added quickly, then recited an address and hung up before I could say more.

It was not a lot of money—a hundred and sixty-two dollars—but there was a principle involved.

I played with the scrap of paper that lay before me, with the hastily scribbled address that the insurance clerk had blurted out. They wanted a letter. I clicked the mouse of my laptop on "Word." They wanted an appeal. I could do that.

Chapter 23

S HE MARKED THE DATE on the kitchen calendar with a big red circle, underlined it three times and added an exclamation mark for emphasis. September 16th— the end of the hundred days.

By the time August began, though, the surgical masks and the latex gloves that sat beside the porch door were no longer being worn by visitors.

"Never mind with that," my wife yelled whenever she heard someone come into the house and fiddle among the boxes of medical supplies. "You can just come in."

They did not go unused, though. I grabbed a glove each morning before going out to paint a little more of the house. And the masks I used to ward off hay fever whenever I mowed the lawn.

Beefsteak tomatoes ripened, and she tossed aside the rule against uncooked vegetables. "I'll just scrub it really good."

"Well, you're a grown girl." I watched her as she stood beside the kitchen sink.

She scrubbed harder at the tomato, highlighting to me that she felt criticized by my comment.

"I think your doctor is being a bit over–cautious." I smiled at her and she stopped scrubbing the tomato long enough to smile back.

She tested the limits and saw that she came to no harm; one by one the rules were abandoned.

She removed her key chain from where it had hung for three months.

"Driving again?" I asked.

"Dancing school starts today," she explained.

"One of your sisters could take her." I poured water into the coffee machine and plugged it in.

She came toward me, reached around behind my back, and flicked a switch on the front of the coffee machine. "You have to turn it on, too," she said softly. Already bothered by the early morning heat, she pulled the bandanna from her head and tossed it onto the kitchen counter. "They did offer to drive, but I feel like getting out of the house." She flashed me a smile as she rubbed the stubble that barely hid her scalp. "I'll open the car window so I can feel the wind through my hair."

I rubbed her stubble too—her hair was not going to be curly or red this time—and together we watched the coffee pour into the clear glass pot.

"Be careful," I ordered. "You haven't driven for a while."

"Drink your coffee and get to work." She pulled the pot out as the last drips fell, then filled my mug. "You'll be late."

"I've got a seminar today," I explained. "I don't have to be in until nine."

I sat in the back row of the seminar, catering to the feeling of isolation which had been growing in me since my wife's bone marrow transplant. I listened as the instructor and the students discussed optimal portfolios, calculation of beta, investment returns. Was standard deviation of returns a good measurement of risk? Who cared? I didn't care.

A woman entered the conference room and carried a note to the instructor. He looked down at the note, then looked up and called my name.

I raised my hand and the woman brought me the note. "Call this number," she whispered.

I recognized the number as my sister-in-law's. "What did she say?" I whispered back, my mouth suddenly dry, my voice barely audible.

"To call," the woman answered before walking away.

I ran from the room to the hall and waited impatiently for the elevator, not even thinking that the stairs to the lobby— just one floor below—would be faster.

In the lobby, a security guard sat behind a wooden desk, his head tipped back against the wall, the brim of his cap flapping up and down like a loose duck bill as he surveyed the crowd with mild interest.

"Is there a phone?" I asked anxiously.

He pointed back from where I had come. "Behind the elevators."

Behind the elevators. What did that mean? I walked between the two bays of elevators and examined each metal door, looking for a picture of a telephone, a smiling Ma Bell— something—until I reached a solid wall. They were all elevator doors. Then I realized what he had meant—behind the elevators meant the hallway after the elevators. Three elevators opened at once, and I was trapped against the solid wall, cut off while a flood of people disembarked and filled the area. They lingered to discuss lunch plans, plot out future meetings, bar my path.

Out of the way, folks! Heart attack in the making!

The crowd slowly thinned, and I found the phone booth occupied.

I ran back to the security guard. He was trying to touch the brim of his cap with his tongue. Several women lingered to one side, watching the display with coy interest.

"Any other phones?" I cried.

He pointed outside.

"Where?" I asked. "In the street?"

"Across the street," he replied rudely.

I was glad I wouldn't be putting my dime in his phone booth.

There were many phones across the street, and I jumped in front of the first empty one. As I dialed my sister-in-law's number, thoughts raced through my head. Perhaps my wife had a heart attack. I stopped dialing—not while driving, don't let it have happened while driving to dancing school—then entered the last two numbers.

She knew it was me before I spoke. Perhaps there was an urgency in my ring. Maybe an 'um' or an 'er' had escaped my mouth and she picked up on it. Perhaps I had screamed "what's happened!" without realizing it.

"She's okay. She's at the hospital." My sister-in-law spoke in a calm voice, and I relaxed slightly. "There's been a car accident."

A car accident, but my wife was okay.

"What about my daughter?" I yelled into the receiver. What was she hiding from me? Good news first. It's always good news first. What was the bad news? What had happened to my daughter?

I waited an eternity within a second before she replied. "She's fine. She cut her lip, but the paramedics gave her a stuffed animal, and she's playing with it here in front of me on the carpet."

I breathed again.

"I'm afraid the van is totaled," she sighed.

Who cares.

"Mom's at the hospital with her," she continued. "They'll come here after they do some x-rays."

Out-of-network, of course.

I didn't find out whether standard deviation of return was the best measure of risk. I doubted that their view of risk was the same as my view of risk. I doubted that the investment world really understood risk at all.

I waited impatiently in the lobby of North Station, watching a woman as she juggled three children and a package between two arms. By the time I got to my sister-in-law's house, my wife had arrived.

"You're walking a little stiff," I said, kissing her carefully.

"I'm feeling a little stiff." She wanted to smile, but she winced instead. "I'm sorry I wrecked the van, but it wasn't my fault." She handed me the paperwork—the police report, the ambulance papers, numerous hospital forms.

"I'm not worried about the van." I found a receipt from the towing company and noted the address.

"A truck pulled out onto the street and hit me. It really wasn't my fault."

"I'll go look at it," I replied. "Maybe it can be fixed."

I brought the mail into the kitchen and leafed quickly through the items addressed to 'occupant,' pulling out the envelope I had been expecting.

"It's the payment from the truck driver's insurance company," I explained as I opened the envelope and looked at the check, surprised to see that the amount had not been reduced.

"Is it enough?" she asked anxiously.

"Well, it's more than we paid for the van two years ago."

"Maybe we can find another used van." Her earlier reluctance was a faded memory, and she was now a van enthusiast.

"I'll get you something new," I offered. "With air bags this time."

"It wasn't my fault," she replied. "The truck hit me." She rubbed her chest—the sore spot where she had hit the steering wheel.

I walked over to her and kissed her boyish hair. "I know. But I'd like to get you something new."

"They won't give us a car loan because of the bankruptcy."

Sadness was creeping into her voice. I knew what would come next if I didn't choose my words carefully: I've ruined your life.

"Now that we have a mortgage, we can get a car loan," I explained. "We've re-established credit." I looked over at the kitchen calendar and saw that it was still on September. I noted with silent amusement that the sixteenth—so prominently marked with red circles and exclamation marks—had passed without notice. Flipping to October, I ran my finger down the new month. "I get paid this Thursday. That will give us a little extra for a down payment."

I looked through the rest of the mail and found a letter from our medical insurance company.

"What's it say?" she asked.

"They denied the appeal," I answered stoically.

"Oh well."

I read the fine print at the bottom of the page. "There's a review board if I want to appeal the decision."

"Appeal the appeal?" she laughed. "This is getting compli-cated."

"I can write them another letter." I folded up the response and set it on the edge of the counter where I wouldn't forget it when I left for work in the morning.

We went the following weekend to the car dealership to pick up our new vehicle. She had picked out a gray van—a Dodge Caravan. "I'll miss Woody," she said, referring to our old van.

"He was a good van." I pushed some buttons on the dash-board. "This one has air conditioning, though."

"It's October. I think you can turn it off." She held the owner's manual open. The dealership had set the clock to the right time, which was a relief. Setting the time was usually the hardest thing about a new vehicle. She was reading about the spare tire. "They put a full size spare on, didn't they?"

"I assume so," I said. "We paid extra for one." I reached over and patted her knee—a silent request for her to relax—then I shifted into forward.

"What should we name her?" she asked.

Our vehicles' names were never arbitrary. Goldie, the Fire-bird, was gold; Woody had fake wood trim before the truck stripped it off; and Lucy, the Daytona, had been bright red, like Lucille Ball.

I thought for a moment. "How about Gracie?"

"I like it," she replied with a smile. "But we can still go to the mountains when it's hot? Even though we now have air conditioning."

The morning was still and dark. I sat on the porch sipping coffee, rocking, wondering where the summer had gone. I heard the patter of feet, the morning joggers running down the street, stuck in habit as I was—5 A.M. and time to run, needing daylight savings to end and for the sun to rise once more when it should.

It was too dark to paint. The clapboard I could paint in the dark by feel, then touch up any spots I missed when the sun finally rose. But I was working on the dentils now, delicate teeth of creamy yellow with a dark brown background. One slip of the brush and I'd have cavities.

She heard my rocker squeaking against the porch floor and walked to the door, the steam rising off of her morning coffee. "Your light's failing you," she said softly as she looked at the darkened morning sky. "What will you do now?"

I shrugged. "Wait for the sun."

Four spotlights hung from the ladder. It was daylight, so they were no longer turned on as I painted between two dentils.

"Do you think you'll finish before your brother gets here?" She stood beside the ladder, shielding her eyes from the low November sun as she watched me paint.

"I think so. I'm almost done up here, and then there's just the front porch remaining."

"I'd help, but I don't know what sort of chemicals are in the paint."

"You relax," I said.

"My hundred days are up, so it's probably okay, but I'm not sure what's in paint." She looked down at the ground, around her feet, looking for a way to feel useful. "I could hold the ladder for you."

"You just relax," I replied. I put a dab of brown on the final dentil, then made a little flourish with my brush to indicated that I was finished up there.

"I'll hold the ladder while you climb down."

Our daughter stood among the rhododendrons splashing white primer on the lattice beneath the porch. She watched me as I stepped off the last rung and onto the grass. "Do we get to do color now?"

"Yes, Pumpkin."

"Are you sure you'll finish in time?" my wife asked, trailing behind me as I carried the can of brown paint toward the porch. "Your brother will be here tomorrow, and we still haven't picked up the turkey." She slowed her pace as she spotted our daughter in the shadow of the largest rhododendron, wiping her hands across her sweatshirt, marking it with broad white streaks. My wife grimaced when she saw the white primer highlighting the little girl's long hair.

"It's latex," I pointed out. "It should wash out."

The little girl trotted over and peeked into the can that dangled from my fingers. "Brown. Yes!" She dipped her paint brush in, leaving a white ring on the surface of the brown paint. "I'm going to paint bunnies, Dada." She ran back beside her favorite shrub and began brushing the brown paint into the white.

My wife grimaced again. "I thought the lattice was going to be sage?"

"I'll fix it later," I whispered.

The sun was still up when I splashed the last stroke of sage across a brown bunny-like object. My daughter had abandoned painting to stand beneath a lilac bush and pretend she was a weatherman.

"Tomorrow, sunny with a chance of berries!" She threw a handful of holly berries into the air. "And that is today's weather news." She placed her arm across her stomach and bowed.

I set my brush in a bucket of warm water and clapped softly.

"Are you done?" She ran to where I stood, leaned close to

the lattice and stared at where her bunnies had been, but said nothing about their disappearance.

"Almost." I took a felt-tipped marker from my shirt pocket. "We just have to sign our names." I pointed to a board that hung beneath the lip of the porch floor—it was cream, a color that would make a good background for the black marker. "You go first."

She printed her name, each letter a little smaller than the one before. When she finished, I took the marker from her hand and scribbled my name beneath hers, then added the year— 1994.

My wife had come out to watch the signing ceremony. "It's a work of art," she proclaimed. "Will you keep the house the same colors next time you have to paint it, or will you go back to one color?"

I looked at her smiling mischievously at me.

"I'll worry about that when the time comes," I laughed, then capped the marker and stuffed it back into my shirt pocket.

Done!

Chapter 24

※

Y WIFE STOOD watching the snow fall
through the parlor window. "Yuck. Winter."

I turned to my wife and asked, "You want to go to Florida
for New Years?"

She nodded.

"It always rains in Florida," I reminded her.

"We'll go anyway," she sighed. "Perhaps it will be a warm
rain."

"Should we bring your mother?" I asked.

She nodded. "Of course."

We landed in Jacksonville and drove to St. Augustine,
where we visited my aunts again. For three days, we were
stuck in the fog. At times, the sun made a valiant effort, dis-
persing the fog just enough so that we could see the barrier

island as we sat on my aunts' dockside porch and sipped coffee. Then it was time to go.

"Daaaahlings, you're leaving us so soon? But you just got here."

"We have to," I explained. "We have reservations in Orlando."

"It's the weather, isn't it?" my elder aunt sighed. "December is always risky."

"It's January," my younger aunt corrected her.

"January is risky, too. Come back in May. May is nice."

"We will," I promised as we waved good-bye through the fog from the car's open window.

We headed inland on a less traveled route that brought us to Orlando via Cross Creek. My wife had chosen that route so we could stop at the home of Marjorie Kinnan Rawlings, author of *The Yearling,* a favorite book of both ours.

We pulled into the dirt parking lot at the Rawlings homestead. As if on cue, the clouds parted and the sun came out—a bit of literary illumination.

A young man in a straw hat greeted us as we ambled down the informal path that led from the parking lot to the Rawlings house. We were in a small orchard that smelled of citrus.

"House is closed today," he said. "The curator didn't show up, and he's got the key. But you can peek in the windows if you like."

We smiled. "Thank you."

"Stop back here on your way out," he said. "Pick yourself some oranges." He handed one he had already picked to our daughter.

She thanked him, then scurried down the path.

The man leaned on his rake and watched as we followed after her, toward a tin roof that peeked out from behind the orchard. "Look as long as you want," he yelled.

A young couple stood on Miss Rawlings' front porch, their

faces pressed against the glass of the parlor window. They turned and left quickly when they heard us approaching, perhaps feeling silly staring through windows, thinking it an odd way to view history and culture.

We took over the young couple's spot and pressed our faces against the glass.

"What do you see?" I asked.

My wife scanned the interior of the room, the few pieces of furniture, the bare walls. "That she was poor."

"Maybe she was eccentric," I suggested.

"No. She was poor."

It was a bit of a shock—the author of *The Yearling* had been poor. She had owned a car—it was still in the carport, license plate and all, as if she were not dead at all, but would come back soon to find us peeking in her windows.

My wife and I looked through another set of windows while my mother-in-law sat in the shade of a lilac, working with my daughter to peel the orange. Seeing the two of them together made me smile.

"Looks like her bedroom," my wife remarked as she peeked through another window.

"Maybe she wasn't poor," I said. "Maybe her relatives came and took most of her stuff when she died."

"Come on," my wife laughed. "Let's leave before you get sunstroke."

On the way out, we each took an orange. I felt guilty taking oranges from a poor lady, even if she were dead, and stuffed another two dollars in the donation box that greeted visitors on their way in.

"I bet she gave her money away to help her neighbors," I suggested. "Or maybe she used her money to start a school for bayou children or something."

We drove down the road toward Orlando. Clouds rolled back across the sky, blotting out the sun.

The next day it didn't rain, but it was cloudy and cool. We did our best to avoid the spray of the motorboats as they raced around the manmade lagoon at Universal Studios.

"Do you want to go on the Jaws ride?" I asked my daughter.

She didn't respond, but looked at me with wide eyes as if I were a madman.

"Don't be silly," my wife said. "She was frightened at the Hanna-Barbera show, and that was a cartoon."

"Well, it was 3-D," I replied. "That can be pretty startling."

We walked past the sign to the Earthquake ride, but I didn't say anything about it to our daughter. There was a playground nearby and she wanted to go there.

"We didn't pay a hundred bucks so you could play on a slide," I complained.

She began to cry. She had a repertoire of fake tears, though I never knew why she bothered with them. I could always recognize them as fake and would chant, "fake tears, fake tears," until she laughed. But these were her real tears. Or perhaps she had perfected her craft.

"Okay, play on the slide. I'll stay here and watch you," I said, and sent my wife and mother-in-law to bicycle off into space with E.T.

The weather was no better along the coast. The town may have been named Clearwater, but that had no effect on the sky.

"I thought this hotel was supposed to be beach front?" My wife held my hand as she spoke.

While her mother unpacked in her room and our daughter played with her latest stuffed animal on our bed, she stood beside me on the balcony looking out at the gray water, the racing white caps, and the wind scouring the beach with sand.

"That's what they said," I replied.

"But there's a highway running between us and the beach," she noted.

I looked down at the traffic running beneath our feet. "I guess the crosswalk makes it beach front."

"We could go to Busch Gardens tomorrow," my wife suggested, seeing, as I did, that it was not going to be beach weather for several days, at least.

Busch Gardens was also cloudy and cool. We rode the flume, getting wet despite the cheap raincoats purchased at the last minute from a souvenir stand. We shivered the rest of the day from our foolishness.

"We'll head south," I suggested. "To Venice. There's a nice beach there where you can find sharks' teeth."

We had not seen the sun for six days now, and it was beginning to irritate me. I had worked all year for this vacation. There seemed something too deliberate about this weather, a cruel joke from the gods. But there was no one to get angry at, and that made it more frustrating. There was no one I could stand before and vent my rage.

"But we're still having fun," my wife pointed out. She scooped a potato chip into a bowl of onion dip and placed it in my mouth.

"I suppose," I said, pausing to chew.

We sat in chairs in our hotel room, facing the water, protected from the elements by a siding glass door. The wind had picked up, and the blowing sand now reached to the top floor of the hotel.

"You saw manatees," she recalled.

"That's true. I saw manatees. In a fish tank."

"They weren't in a fish tank." She stroked my hair and kissed gently at my ear.

"No. We were in the fish tank." I frowned at the grayness of the sky and the sea before us, a bit jealous that the manatees were free to swim, but I had been dry-docked by the weather.

"See?" she laughed. "You got to go in a fish tank."

I laughed, too. "You're right. It's just nice to be away." I kissed her, leaving a bit of onion dip where our lips had touched. "We'll head south tomorrow, to Venice, and hunt for sharks' teeth."

"What makes you think there's sharks' teeth in Venice?" she asked.

"My grandparents lived there when I was a boy," I explained. "That's what we did on our winter vacations. Hunted sharks' teeth." I described to her how my brothers and I stood watching the waves break, spotting the sharks' teeth with our eager young eyes as they rolled about in the surf, and how the sand tickled our feet as the waves hurled themselves upon the beach. I described what I thought was a romantic image—Norman Rockwell, perhaps—but I looked at her and saw she did not have the faraway look of someone caught up in my fond memory. She looked alarmed.

"Are there sharks, too?" she asked anxiously.

"No," I said calmly. "Just teeth."

"I would think wherever there were sharks' teeth there would be sharks," she said, still worried.

"They're fossil teeth," I said. "They're from prehistoric sharks."

She glanced at me with her dubious look, but she agreed to go. "Only because you're not having fun here," she said.

We drove south, out of Clearwater and away from the pawn shops and strip malls. Away from the girlie shows and the T-shirt shops. Past the Ringling Brothers' Circus museum, past the billboards advertising the World's greatest basket shop. The clouds did not lift, but the air warmed some. It was not warm enough for my wife or mother-in-law, though, so my daughter and I ran down to the beach alone, leaving the two women sitting in the car behind the sand dunes.

On the beach, despite the clouds, retirees sifted the wet sand with screen boxes attached to broom handles. A mechanized search for the elusive sharks' teeth. The world had become a more sophisticated place since I was a boy. Back then, you looked for sharks' teeth by standing in the surf and grabbing them with your bare hand as they tumbled between your feet. Now equipment was required.

The water had become too cloudy. It was not the clear water of my youth, and now I could barely see my toes. I grabbed random handfuls of sand as the waves crashed around me, bringing up nothing but sand and rock until—pay dirt.

"Here's a shark's tooth!" I held it up excitedly. "See?" I had beaten out the retirees and found one with my bare hands. The simple ways of my youth were still the best.

My daughter looked quickly at the tooth, then turned away and picked up a broken scallop shell.

I grabbed more sand. It had been a little tooth. Perhaps a bigger one would impress her. "Here's another tooth." I handed it to my daughter, but she was more interested in the scallop shell she had found. I gathered three teeth together, then we returned to the car.

"You can still find them," I said to my wife, and dropped the teeth into her hand. "The water's a lot cloudier than when we were kids, though."

"From the rain?" she asked.

"No, from too much development."

My wife held a tooth up close to her eye. "They're not very big. I thought prehistoric sharks were large."

"There are bigger ones," I said. "But the water's too cloudy."

In the back seat, my mother-in-law examined one of the teeth herself, but said nothing.

We never did see the Florida sun. A sense of failure accompanied me as we returned home. But it was my fault: I knew that if we went to Florida it would rain, and I went anyway.

Chapter 25

༄

I ENTERED THE HOUSE with a letter in one
hand and a grocery bag stuffed with mail in the other hand,
pushing the porch door open with my shoulder.

"What's wrong?" My wife spotted the shadows creasing
my face the moment I stepped into the kitchen.

"I got a reply from the insurance company." I held up the
lone letter as I set the grocery bag on the kitchen counter.
"They denied my appeal."

A large pile of mail had accumulated at the post office while
we were away. I had gone alone to pick it up, and set it on the
front seat beside me, sifting through it with my free hand as I
steered the van homeward. I spotted the letter as my eyes
darted back and forth between the mail and the street, lying

there beside the K-mart flyer, and knew that the appeal had been denied.

"Oh well," she said, spreading the contents of the grocery bag across the counter. "You tried."

"I'm not done yet." I was about to crumple the letter into a little ball and toss it into the waste basket, but thought better of it. Evidence. I would need it for the next step.

"What can you do now?" She did not look at me as we spoke, but went about sorting the mail into three piles—hers, mine, and junk. She held up an advertisement with my name on it. "You want this?"

"No." I took it from her and crumpled it, tossing it into the trash, a proxy for the one I wished to crumple. "I'll go to the State Insurance Office," I said. "That's what I'll do."

"It's not a lot of money."

"No," I said. "But we had a deal. They said if you went to their hospital, they'd pay the whole bill."

She conveyed her agreement by the shortness of her silence. A long silence would have meant she disagreed. "What would you like for dinner?"

"Fish?" I answered, watching her sort the mail. Her pile was fun—magazines, sales brochures, a letter from a far-off sister-in-law.

"Not fish," she groaned, and tossed another bill onto my pile.

"Spaghetti?"

"Okay."

She left the mail for me to finish sorting through and stepped toward the cabinet where we kept the large pots. "It's not a lot of money, you know," she said as she pulled down her favorite spaghetti pot. "It's not worth getting all worked up over."

"No, but there's a principle involved."

She looked out the window as she ran water into the pot. "It's starting to snow."

I came up behind her and set my chin on her shoulder. Together we looked out at the gently falling snow.

"So it is," I said softly.

Then we were silent.

"You're thinking of skiing, aren't you?" She turned away and carried the pot to the stove. "You two can go. I'll stay here."

"I was thinking of Canada. Shopping in Montreal. Hot cocoa at Mont-Tremblant."

She was facing away from me, and I studied her shoulders for a reaction.

"Do you still want to stay behind?" I asked.

She turned back and smiled at me. "You don't play fair, do you?"

"Never," I smirked. "Just ask the insurance company."

"Don't you look smug," she remarked as I strolled into the kitchen and kissed her neck.

She noticed right off: the way I tossed my coat onto the coat hook rather than draping it; the way I inhaled the aroma of her homemade onion soup—"Ahhhh."

"Get a raise or something?" she asked.

"Without you? Never," I quipped as I dipped the ladle into the pot for a quick taste of her soup, but she grabbed it from my hand before I could get my lips on it. "I went down to the State Insurance Office the other day."

"You told me already," she remarked dryly.

"And who do you think called me this afternoon?" I waited for a reply, but grew impatient watching as she seasoned the soup. "The lady from the insurance company. The one who likes to deny appeals."

"Oh?" There was only mild interest in her voice. She picked up a chunk of gruyere and began grating it into the three soup bowls.

"They reconsidered my appeal and agreed to pay me the hundred and sixty-two dollars." I waited for some applause or something, but there was only the sound of cheese being grated. "She didn't even mention the State Insurance Office. Acted like she went ahead and did it on her own, like she had done me a big favor."

"Whatever," my wife replied blandly. "At least you got your money."

"I wanted to say something rude to her," I continued, hoping to get more of a response from her, "like 'Well, it's about time, you ignorant slut.' But instead I said, 'Thank you.'"

"That's always best," she said. "You come out looking better for it."

"She said we should get the check by the end of the month," I said, my voice trailing off as I realized the money was of little interest to her.

"Maybe we'll have it in time for Montreal." She lifted the ladle toward my lips, and I slurped the soup eagerly.

We waited until President's Day Weekend to go to Montreal. That means nothing to the Canadians—just another weekend—so the crowds that would be swarming around the ski lifts south of the border would be nonexistent to the north.

We left without the check from the insurance company. Next month, they said. The paperwork hadn't cleared in time for this month.

"Look for a big cheese grater." My wife held a guide book open in her lap, trying not to look down at it for too long. She could never read in the car without getting sick, and since her treatments, had found the situation even worse.

"A cheese grater?" Our daughter giggled from the back seat. She had been good for the past six hours, though we had to listen to "She'll be comin' round the mountain" eighteen times on the cassette player. She wanted to hear it a nineteenth time, but I said no. She sulked then, remaining silent in the back seat, except to talk quietly with her invisible sisters, the three of them plotting against the adult world. But now that we were in Montreal, she forgot her anger and was talking again. "Why do we want a cheese grater?"

"The hotel looks like a big cheese grater, dear," my wife explained. "That's what the guide book says, anyway."

"Can I take a right turn on red?" I asked.

"I have no idea," my wife replied, leafing quickly through the book as if the answer were somewhere in there.

"Probably not," I assumed. "Canadians are more patient than Americans."

"Canadians say they are Americans," she noted.

"They're North Americans," I argued, "not Americans."

Her finger darted toward the left and touched the windshield. "There!" She pulled her finger away, leaving a smudge on the glass. "The cheese grater."

The next day, we drove to the top of Mount Royal to get a view of Montreal. A woman came from nowhere and started talking to me in French before I even knew she was there.

"I'm sorry," I replied. "I don't understand French."

I wanted to explain that I had nearly flunked French in the sixth grade and had switched quickly to German, but she threw her hands in the air and stormed off, shouting out an eloquent stream of French insults.

"I didn't know they hated Americans here," my wife whispered.

"I didn't either." I watched the woman as she walked past our van, her eyes darting down toward our license plate. Her face suddenly brightened and she smiled. She spun around and strolled back.

"I am sorry, monsieur, but the parking booth at that end is closed," she said sweetly, acting as though the prior incident had never occurred. "You will have to go to the other one to pay."

"Merci," I replied, quickly thinking that the merci was a mistake, that perhaps she'd think I was not entirely honest about my lack of French.

She smiled smugly—she could tell by my poor pronunciation that I had not lied about my French. Then she sauntered off.

"What was that all about?" my wife asked.

"She saw our license plate and came back," I explained. "I guess it's just their own countrymen they don't like."

"Would monsieur and madame like a sleigh ride?" A smallish woman with a manly way sat in a sleigh behind two horses. She tried to smile, but the effort looked painful.

I looked at my wife and she nodded back.

"Oh, and you have a little one," the woman said, smiling this time.

She helped us into the back of the sleigh and wrapped us in scratchy blankets. Clicking her tongue softly, the sleigh lurched forward, moving us swiftly up the hill along the same path used by pedestrians. Bells jingled from the horses' necks, sending people scurrying from the path and into the snowy fields.

I thought several times that we would run over those who did not react quickly enough to the sound of the bells, but the horses were well-trained and would stop without a command from the driver. Then they would walk slowly along, tossing their necks and ringing their bells loudly until the people moved to one side and the horses could jog once again.

"Do you like our city?" the driver turned around and asked, frowning.

"It's lovely," my wife replied. "It's very clean."

The woman jiggled the reins just enough to let the horses know that she was there. "I go to Florida sometimes," she said.

This time I frowned.

"Sometimes winter is just too long." She stopped the sleigh. "You can get out here and walk to the stone wall. You get a good view there."

I helped my wife and daughter from the sleigh.

"Two minutes," the driver said. "I give you two minutes." She held her watch up to show us she would know if we went over our allotted time.

Beneath us was a city draped in winter. Unlike American cities, buttoned up against the cold, people scowling at the first snowflake of each storm, Montreal knew how to enjoy winter. Off in the distance, along the waterfront, were the final scenes of a company picnic—ice skating, a children's playground crafted from snow, the smoke from a barbecue pit. How many American companies would hold their employee outing in the dead of winter?

The sun shone brightly that day, slowly melting the snow, water dripping from the rooftops of the outbuildings as we stood at the peak of Mount Royal. Hordes of people climbed toward us, laughing and smiling, their bright red and blue coats a colorful display against the white snow and the gray trees. Younger children pushed one another into snow banks, enjoying a weekend outing, not avoiding snow like it was acid, but instead hunting out the remaining patches and strolling across them as though they were fine carpets. A thousand feet were crunching, crunching throughout the park, like a house full of hungry termites.

"I think our two minutes is up." My wife turned me gently around and pointed toward the sleigh.

In the distance, I could see our driver tapping her watch impatiently, her hardened face scowling further. Perhaps I had been wrong. Perhaps Canadians are Americans after all.

We woke up early the next morning and left the cheese grater, heading north toward the Laurentians. The road to Mont-Tremblant was lined with ski areas; I had never seen so many in one place. Even my wife, now a non-skier, was overwhelmed by the spectacle.

"How do they all stay in business?" she asked.

"Canadians like to ski," I explained.

Further into the mountains we went until we were shrouded in fog. We missed our turn—or rather, we made a turn we shouldn't have—and came out on the back side of Mont-Tremblant, at an area with only limited facilities.

"You go ski," she said. "I'll be fine here."

"No," I insisted. "We'll drive around to the other side. There should be someplace for you to sit there."

The delay cost us—the children's ski school had already left for the slopes, so I enrolled our daughter in a private class with a handsome Frenchman named Jacque instead. While I tended to our daughter, my wife sat among the clutter of the lower ski lodge, an area dominated by wooden benches and devoid of comfort.

"Why are you sitting down here?" I asked after leaving our daughter with Jacque.

"Where else should I go?"

I took her hand and led her to a little gondola, then pointed up the slope. "There's a cute village up there."

"Don't take me up the mountain. Please."

I kissed her cheek. "It's just a little way, honey. You could walk it if you wanted to, but this way is easier."

The ride was short, as I had promised, and at the other end was an alpine village with chocolate shops, gift boutiques, taverns, cafes, and a T-shirt shop.

"It is cute," she observed.

The ground fog had lifted, but the upper reaches of the mountain were still encased in a thick white cloud, giving the mountain an odd truncated look, like a volcano.

"You're going up there?" she asked.

"We've come all this way," I explained.

"Be careful," she warned. "You're skiing alone."

I kissed her and said good-bye, then said good-bye to the sunshine and climbed aboard the chair lift for the ride to the top.

I skied alone, lost in a white void, an occasional gray hobgoblin gliding silently past in the mist. My eyes were like the eyes of sleep, squinting, but seeing nothing real—vague images, ghosts. I lost myself in the whiteness, not knowing whether my skis carried me downhill to safety or uphill to remain lost forever in the clouds.

Suddenly, bright light appeared. Out of the fog and into life. And far below, the pretty village, with people looking like ants, sitting around tiny tables with green and blue umbrellas, sipping drinks. And somewhere—my wife.

"Are you going back up after lunch?" she asked.

"Too much fog," I answered. "It gives me vertigo." I pointed to our daughter, sitting beside my wife and happily slurping a Shirley Temple. "I'll take her up the bunny slope instead."

We returned that night to the cheese grater. In the morning we packed our bags and headed for home, avoiding the expressways, taking the slow way through quiet French villages that dotted the snowy plains above Lake Champlain.

"Why do you think more Americans don't visit Canada?" I asked.

"Canadians are Americans," my wife replied.

Chapter 26

*S*HE WAS STANDING by the porch door, waiting anxiously for me to return home from work.

"What are you hiding from me?" she screamed as she
watched me climb the stairs.

I looked at her with genuine confusion. "Nothing. Why?"

"The oncology department called me," she explained, her
voice shrill with anxiety. "They said they needed to change
your appointment."

Uh oh. Plot uncovered.

I had gone for my annual checkup. There was a minor
problem with my blood counts. Nothing to worry about, my
doctor said, but he wanted it checked out by a hematologist,
just to be safe.

I didn't tell my wife—I knew how she'd worry. Who could
know that the hematologist's wife would go into labor two

weeks early, and he'd have to cancel my appointment? They called my office and left a message, but apparently they called my wife, too, just to make sure I got the message.

"We'll joke about this some day," I said nervously as I set my briefcase down and kissed her gently on her lips, the way I always did. Nothing special, see? No cause for alarm.

"We'll joke about what?" she asked, staring at me with eyes wide, terror showing that she had never shown through her own ordeal. "Why are you seeing an oncologist?"

"Not an oncologist," I corrected her. "A hematologist."

"Same thing," she replied, her eyes getting so big and white, she was beginning to scare me. "What's wrong?"

"My white blood counts are a bit high." I took her shoulders between my palms, and looked her straight in the eyes. "There's nothing wrong."

"Then why did you hide it from me?" She wanted to pace, but I held her so she couldn't.

"I didn't want you to worry," I explained.

"Well, now I am," she cried. "If you had told me, I wouldn't have."

She would have, but I didn't say that. Frankly, I was a bit worried myself. My mother had a high white blood count, and then she died.

I anxiously waited three days while the hematologist bonded with his newborn son. He returned to work, his eyes dark from a lack of sleep.

"How's the baby?" I asked.

He looked at me from across his desk—young, wealthy, handsome in a skinny, intellectual way—and smiled. "Fine." He held out a small snapshot of a pink baby hidden in a white blanket, a blue knit cap pulled down below his eyebrows. "You have any children?"

"One," I said. "A girl."

For a moment we pretended we were more to each other than doctor and patient, then he took out a pad, breaking the spell. He scratched a rude diagram of veins and blood cells, explaining to me how most white blood cells were normally attached to the walls of the veins, how sometimes they just decided to hop off and ride around in the bloodstream for awhile for no reason, just to cause us alarm.

"Don't be alarmed, though," he assured me. "I see this all the time."

"Will I get better?" I asked.

"You aren't sick," he replied.

I wasn't sick. My blood cells were just out for a joyride, and I was their anxious parent waiting for them to come home.

The doctor ordered a few tests, just to be safe, but I never heard from him again. When I found myself alive and well a year later, I stopped worrying about my high white blood count. I assumed all my little children had come home to roost, that they were clinging somewhere under my armpit for now, but on some future date they'd all hop off again and go for another spin.

My regular physician marked my chart, indicating that a high white count was normal for me.

Twelve little girls dressed in white lace danced across the stage, then stopped. In the middle was our daughter, kneeling, waiting patiently for the fairy princess to tap her head with the magic wand and send her gently spinning toward the audience.

There were real dance steps now. Not like the prior year: a morass of arm movements and chanting voices; a few pointed toes; and chubby-faced toddlers scratching most unladylike at their panties. This year, their growing feet moved in patterns that indicated that a complex dance step had been learned.

Their movements were no longer identical—one girl would spin right, another would spin left. One poor girl wouldn't spin at all and ran crying into the side curtain to find comfort in the arms of an older girl waiting there in the wings. A hush fell over the crowd—we all felt for the girl as though she was our own. Such a fragile age.

Tears formed in my eyes, just as they had the year before, and I looked over at my wife and wondered—how long?

I squeezed her knee, and she smiled timidly back at me, her thoughts joined with my thoughts—how long?

The lights came on, the show was over. Another year. Another precious year. A gift.

I looked about and saw the emptiness of the auditorium, a room that had been overflowing three hours earlier.

"Where is everyone?" I asked.

"Most people go home after their child dances," my wife explained, then dropped her voice to a whisper. "Help me up, please."

"Are you okay?" I asked, concerned by her sudden weakness.

She nodded slowly.

I held my hand out to her. "That seems rude, walking out on a show."

She shrugged. "It does, doesn't it. I guess three hours is too long for some people to sit."

"Do you think they walk out on football games, too?"

"Maybe if their team is losing." She smiled, then pulled hard on my arm, trying to lift herself from the seat.

She caught me unprepared, and I tipped toward her. "You sat for too long," I said. "That's why you can't get up."

"No, it's not that," she whispered. "It's come back."

My wife had been complaining for several months about odd pains. After the dance recital, it only got worse. She waited until her normal appointment, then pointed out all her sore spots once more to her doctor.

"Still have that pain in the back?" her doctor asked.

"And the hip," she explained.

He leafed through the thick folder that held my wife's records, a synopsis of the past four years of her life. "The tumor marker was normal last time, and there was nothing on your last x-rays." He flipped through the final pages, looking for when the last bone scan had been done, then counted the months off on his finger. "It's been six months," he said. "We should do another bone scan. And another tumor marker."

Early the next morning, we drove with the rush hour crowd—there was no way to avoid the Boston traffic when a bone scan was needed. She checked in at outpatient registration, then signed in again at radiology.

We sat together and read old magazines, watching, a bit confused, as an attendant in green scrubs led latecomers in before us.

"They should at least give me my shot while we're sitting here," she said. "I have to wait three hours after that before they can do the scan."

Forty-five minutes later, I went to the receptionist to see where we stood on their list.

"Sit down," she ordered. "We'll call you."

Forty-five minutes after that, I went to the receptionist again.

She was indignant, but she phoned the secret room in back, a place where I envisioned idle x-ray technicians stood around devouring donuts and slurping coffee, unseen by the general public.

"What do you mean, you didn't know she was here? She's on the list out here!" She slammed down the receiver and switched to her charm school face. "I'm sorry, but they neglected to tell the nurse that you were here."

I stared at her, saying nothing, letting my gaze linger on her until she looked away uncomfortably, staring down at her own breasts, wondering if perhaps a button had come loose.

I smiled, mouthed a thank you, and returned to my wife's side. "We must have a kick me sign on our butts," I said as I snatched the magazine from my chair.

It was four hours more before my wife was done. Then we waited upstairs on wooden chairs in the hallway outside her doctor's office. Waited with sweaty hands while downstairs the bone pictures were developed, and her doctor examined them with the radiologist.

I heard him coming up the back staircase, the one marked "emergency only." We were an emergency. His feet were heavy, plodding, as he burst through the door and into the hallway.

"Come with me," he said softly.

We rose quickly and followed him to the examination room.

He slipped the films into the view box and switched on its light, then studied the little skeletons that hung before him. "There's one on the thoracic spine, and another one below that." He didn't point them out this time—she knew better than the doctors where they were. "And it looks like there's one on your hip bone."

"See," she said. "That's just where I've been saying they were." Triumph. Body and mind over hard science, but she was not rejoicing. "That's all my sore spots."

"Tumors aren't normally painful," her doctor explained, a meek way of apologizing for not believing my wife sooner.

"Mine are," she replied.

"From now on, we'll just skip all the high-tech tests," I threatened. "We'll let her tell us where the tumors are."

"Fair enough," her doctor replied, not offended by what I said. "There could be some truth in what you're saying."

He studied the films again, not looking for anything undiscovered—the radiologist had already pointed out all the hot spots for him—but more to remind himself of what the radiologist had said. "There's at least two tumors in the spine." He referred to them in code, calling them C-7, C-9, or some such nonsense. Then he picked up my wife's folder. "Obviously, we can't do another bone marrow transplant. Your bone marrow has been too weakened for that."

"Could she do chemo again?" I asked hopefully.

He looked through her charts and tallied up her lifetime of drug dosages. "She can't do Adriamycin. She's had her limit of that. But she can do 5-FU again, if we keep the dosage low."

My wife sat silent and let the men do the talking this time. She was tired and no longer trusted her thoughts.

"She should start right away," he explained.

"Today?" I asked.

"No," my wife interrupted. "I want to go away."

Yes! Finally! Join me. Run. We'll run away together.

"For a week." She looked at me, her eyes begging. "Can we take one last vacation?"

"Okay. But then you have to come back here for treatment," I replied.

"Then I'll be dead," she said quietly.

"No." I took her hand and squeezed it gently. "You'll live to be a hundred."

Her doctor wanted to start right away, to get to work on those tumors before they did any serious damage, but he also knew—or tried to envision—what my wife had gone through the past four years. "All right," he said. "We'll start in two weeks. Go someplace warm, rest up, and I'll see you in two weeks."

Chapter 27

*T*HE THREE OF US boarded a charter flight for Aruba. Last minute tickets, bargain basement prices.

"This is the way to do it," I remarked happily as I watched the flight attendant direct our attention to the overhead screens. "If you don't care where you're going."

"Most people like to know where they're heading before they start packing." My wife smiled, amused by my cheapness, relieved that the charter plane had a modern look.

"It wasn't that bad," I said. "I got the tickets four days ago."

June, and the flight was filled with newlyweds. A young bride smiled at us. She smiled at our daughter, imagining her own family, soon to be created. Two, maybe three, she'd have.

Other smiling brides turned in their seats when they heard the voice of the chatty four-year-old beside me. Our daughter smiled back at them, not fully understanding their peculiar smirks.

In less time than it took to get a bone scan, we were whisked from the troubled spring of Boston to the tropical breezes of Aruba.

"It's nice to feel the heat," my wife said as we lounged together in a hammock under a palm tree. "I don't know what happened to our spring this year."

"Your back doesn't hurt?" I asked, concerned more with her than the Boston weather.

"A little," she replied. "When you rock us too hard."

I stopped rocking the hammock, but the palm trees continued to sway in the stiff trade winds; and looking up into the fluttering palm fronds, the sensation of movement was still there.

I looked toward the sea. "I could take you out on the air mattress. You'll be safe with me."

"Not too far, though," she replied sternly.

"To the inside of the coral reef, so you can see the fish."

She was frightened as I pushed her and the inflated air mattress into deeper water.

"There were two reef squid out here earlier," I remarked as I clung to the back of the mattress.

"Oh?" she replied, too frightened to say more.

We heard an indistinct shout and looked toward shore. A head bobbed half-way between us and the sandy beach, and we saw that it was our daughter.

"I'm coming to save you, Mommy!"

"But she can't swim that far," my wife gasped, and started paddling her arms, turning the mattress toward the lone head bobbing in the surf. She began kicking, then stopped and stretched her neck upwards, trying to see over the rolling sea as the little head disappeared between two waves.

The head appeared again. I could see the flash of orange against either cheek. "She's okay," I shouted. "She's got her water wings on."

"I'm coming, Mommy!" she called again, and switched from doggy paddle to an odd form of breaststroke. "I'll . . . save . . . you."

"Let's go back and get her anyway," my wife said, anxiety rising in her voice.

"She's fine," I replied.

"She could lose a water wing or something." My careless attitude did not anger her. She was merely worried for our daughter. "Who's going to keep her safe when I'm gone?"

"Then you better not leave us," I threatened playfully. I told her that often, every time I did something stupid. Sometimes I did things that were stupid—burn the toast, mix colors and whites in the washer—just so she could she how badly we needed her.

I snagged the air mattress by its rope handle and swam toward our daughter. As we reached her, she grabbed the rope. "I'm saving you, Mommy."

And she was. Not from drowning, but from the more immediate danger that had followed my wife, living in her shadow for four long years.

Once again I picked up the mail at the post office. This time there was no letter from the insurance company, but there should have been. There should have been a check for one hundred and sixty-two dollars. It had been five or six months since they told the State Insurance office that they would reimburse me.

I called the claims office and got the appeals lady on the phone.

"I'm waiting for approval from my supervisor," she explained tersely.

"For six months?" I asked, fighting to contain my exasperation.

"Five months," she argued.

"Five months to get a signature?" I chided.

"My supervisor is waiting for some paperwork from the home office."

"Never mind." I hung up.

My wife hovered nearby. "What are you going to do now?" she asked.

"Change tactics," I replied. "Remember last year? I told you that I met one of the insurance company's presidents at a seminar."

"Yes, I remember."

"I mentioned that you had breast cancer, and it turned out his first wife had died from breast cancer."

"I remember you telling me that," she replied, her voice vague, indicating she was not entirely sure where I was going with this.

"I bet if I write him a letter and tell him how the benefits people are treating us, he'll do something."

"Just be careful what you say," she warned. "Don't get fired over a hundred bucks."

I was diplomatic. I explained that I had been waiting six months—maybe five—for a check that did not seem to be forthcoming, and that since his wife had been a victim of the same disease that my wife now suffered from, perhaps he could relate to the horror we were going through and use his influence to get the check issued.

Bam! Did I hit the right button.

Three days later the President of Group Benefits called to say he was sorry about the delay, and the check was in the mail. Ten minutes after that, the head supervisor in Kalamazoo called to say she was very sorry, and the check was in the mail. Five minutes after that, the appeals lady called to say she was a little sorry. She didn't know if the check was in the mail because she was just the appeals lady. They must have had one big meeting about my wife, and once it was over, hurried to their phones, trying desperately to get the heat turned down.

"He knows the President!" they shouted through the halls. "Damn! He knows the President!"

That's what you have to do with insurance companies, just keep pushing their buttons until you hit the right one. My wife was ill; I couldn't help her there, but I could sit at my desk and push the insurance company's buttons. That was something I could do. It was my therapy.

We walked together down the cancer center's familiar hall, between the elegant columns of what had once been a grand mansion. The cuckoo clock at the end of the hall struck eleven-thirty even though it was ten-fifteen. It wasn't working the first time we were there. That was four years ago. They still hadn't fixed it. They hadn't fixed my wife, either. What had they been doing for four years? What had all the cancer researchers been doing all those years? Four years, and here we were, back in the cancer center, and here was 5-FU still waiting for us.

The nurse was expecting us. As we entered the treatment room, I spotted the fanny pack, the needles, the gauze lying on a table, spread out like a salesman's display. They were on the same table as three years before. My wife sat down in the large brown chair, and I instinctively rolled the little blue office chair from out of the corner and to a spot beside her. Déjà vu. Yes, we had done all this before.

The nurse tugged the white curtain along its tracks, providing us with a bit of privacy. We had been doing this for so long, we rarely thought of privacy anymore, but the nurse still did.

She let go of the curtain and sat down beside my wife, feeling my wife's portacath with her fingertips, learning the setup before proceeding, then swabbing my wife's collar bone with iodine, or something that looked like iodine.

"It's still working," the nurse commented as she stuck a syringe into the portacath and drew out a small quantity of blood.

"It will probably be the last thing on me to go," my wife replied. "Archeologists will find a perfectly functional portacath among my crumpled bones."

The nurse smiled, unsure of what type of response was called for. Humor in the halls of death. "Now this is a one week supply," she explained as she attached a plastic bag containing the 5-FU to the little pump and tucked them both inside the fanny pack. "It might look empty before the week is out, but it's not."

My wife nodded. It had been three years, but the instructions were still a vivid memory. The treatment was still a vivid memory, and she wanted to cry.

"How old's your daughter now?" the nurse asked.

Our daughter—a bright spot, and my wife quickly smiled. "Four," she said. "Almost five. She'll be starting kindergarten this fall."

"Kindergarten," the nurse sighed. "That's great." She patted my wife's shoulder. "All set. I'll see you next week."

"I hate this," she cried. "I really really hate this." She sat in the living room, perched in her chair—the mechanized one she had inherited from her father, along with a wheelchair. A pink bath towel hung over her shoulders. She grabbed the two ends, staring down in disgust at the towel's shabbiness. "I thought I told you to throw these out."

Throw these out! She had said that a year ago, maybe. Get some new ones! But they were still there in the bathroom, worn thin, long white strands of thread hanging from their ends. Where had the pink gone? Washed away, I supposed. Years and years of bleach.

"I guess I forgot to," I stammered.

She shook her head, but I saw the grin sneak across her face and knew she was amused. As usual, I amused her with my forgetfulness.

She tightened her grasp on the towel's frayed ends and pulled them around her neck. Hair was going to fall and she didn't want it irritating her neck. "Go ahead. Do it."

I picked up her good sewing scissors and began snipping, watching as her hair fell in bunches onto the pink bath towel. "But it's a good sign, losing your hair again. It means the chemo still works."

"It's killing hair follicles, not cancer," she fumed, keeping her head bowed low so I could get to the hair around the back of her neck.

"But that means it's killing cancer, too."

"No. It's not. It's killing hair, not cancer. I can feel the tumors growing. Every day my body gets a little bit sorer." She began to cry.

I wanted to say "don't cry," but I didn't. She had earned a good cry. If anyone should cry, it was she. I set the scissors on the coffee table and flicked the switch to her chair, starting up the motor and lifting her closer and closer to me. The motor pushed her higher, nearer to me, close enough that the warm breath of her sobs bathed my cheeks. I reached out and pulled her to my chest.

"It's just a waste of time," she sobbed, her tears soaking my shirt. "You should just let me go. Take me to Michigan to that doctor and end it."

"No, you'll get better again," I uttered.

"No," she cried. "I'll never feel better again." Her sobs became louder.

Our daughter poked her head into the room. She had heard her mother crying and wondered what was wrong. But she recognized it for what it was and hurried to the parlor to play, not fully understanding any of it, but knowing it was something she was too young to deal with.

I knew the game she would play there. I had found her in the parlor before, at other times similar to this, curled up in the JC Penny chair, playing "orphan girls" with her invisible sisters. "My mommy's dead." "Well, so is mine," she would chat back and forth using an assortment of amiable voices.

"I'm never going to feel good again," my wife moaned.

"You'll snap back," I replied. "You always snap back. You're my little rubber band." I stroked her head, forgetting about her hair until I felt the strands as they stuck between my fingers, reminding me that my task was not done. "Snap," I said, trying to sound cheerful.

She smiled, enjoying the way I said snap. Her tears began to subside.

I said it once more. "Snip Snap!"

"Yeah, I'll snap all right. I'll snap in half." She eased herself back into her chair, then set the switch into the opposite direction, slowly lowering herself to a sitting position. "Come on. Finish this job," she demanded as she snatched up the sewing scissors and handed them back to me.

Chapter 28

*S*HE LAY BESIDE ME, moaning. Her doctor had prescribed morphine, but she stopped taking it. I had been sleeping facing the wall, but turned to face her as I carefully rubbed her shoulders.

"Why don't you try the morphine again?" I suggested.

"It makes me nauseous," she said. "And my head just swims."

"Does it help the pain?"

"No. Not really," she replied drowsily. "It just makes me so I don't care." She tried to adjust the position of her legs, but the pain was too much. "Could you pull my legs toward you a bit?"

I slid her legs inwards until they touched mine. "Did the Darvon help?"

"Not much."

The Darvon had been a desperate act by her doctor. It didn't have any properties that should cure pain, he said, but for some reason it did help some people. Not my wife, though.

"Do you want to try a Percocet?" I asked, recalling the friend from school who went to jail over Percocets. They had to be good.

"They made me throw up last time." She squirmed slightly. "Maybe another pillow under my left shoulder."

I wedged a pillow beneath her shoulder, moving slowly so as not to jolt her. "I would think you'd prefer nausea over pain."

"It might seem so," she sighed, "but after you've been nauseous for a few days, you prefer the pain."

I fluffed up another pillow and tucked it under her head.

"I hate the night," she complained. "I'd just like to be able to get comfortable again." She began to cry.

I wrapped my arm over her shoulder, and pulled her toward me. Gently. "You will. Soon."

"No," she cried. "The pain will never leave. Only when I die."

"How about a Tylenol?" I suggested.

She nodded her head slightly as it lay against the pillow. "Regular," she said. "Not the codeine ones."

It was late June, but the house seemed cold as I slipped out from under the covers and walked to the bathroom in my bare feet. I stood before the medicine cabinet and stared in at the huge array of drugs. I searched the bottles—codeine, Percocet, morphine, Darvocet, Dilaudid, M S Contin. I found the Tylenol, but kept examining the other bottles and boxes out of morbid curiosity. Opiates in all its forms—pills, skin patches, suppositories, time release capsules. Full strength, half strength, and, finally, quarter strength, but to no avail. Her brain rejected drugs in all their forms.

"You should have practiced drug abuse in college," I had

teased her on more than one occasion. "Then your brain would be used to it."

"Wouldn't a drug addict love to get in this house," I called as I dug further into the pill supply. I had needed my driver's license to fill several of the prescriptions. For one I had to go to a neighboring town—our pharmacist said he didn't carry that drug because it attracted burglars. "You sure you don't want to try the morphine again? Your body might adjust to it if you tried it for a few days."

"Just a Tylenol," she called back.

Zofran—three dollars a pill—to combat nausea. She wasn't nauseous in her stomach, her doctor had explained. She was nauseous in her head. She chased a morphine with the Zofran, but she was still nauseous in the head and in the stomach.

"You want to try the joint?"

She laughed.

A friend at work had given me some pot. He had heard of my wife's predicament and he wanted to help. She wouldn't smoke it, though. It was against the law. I stashed it in the attic with the fireworks she wouldn't let me shoot off.

I brought her one pill—a prescription Tylenol, super-strength, no codeine—and a glass of water. "I could get you some wine. That might help."

"Right." She looked at me, flashing her odd smirk that told me she thought I was pulling her leg.

"No, really. Alcohol is a good pain killer. That's what they would give a pirate before they cut off his leg." I swung my fist through the air as though it held a tankard of rum. "Yo-ho-ho."

"Get back into bed," she said. "I'll fall asleep eventually."

❧

The little pump whirled and whirled without fail, every fifteen minutes, through the nights, the days. 5-FU slowly seeped throughout her system, her body absorbing it like she was a big wet sponge.

"Everything tastes like chemicals." She smacked her lips together and made a sour face.

"Then you won't want to buy too much food," I teased.

We were going grocery shopping. I unfolded the wheelchair, the one that had come from her father's house after he died. I had stashed it in the basement wondering what the hell I would do with a wheelchair. But her blood counts dropped and she weakened, and the only way she could join us now on family outings was in the wheelchair.

She had tried to continue on foot, walking slowly and erect so the pressure of the tumors wouldn't send jolts of pain through her spine. But on the last outing, in the cake mix aisle at the local supermarket, a box of Betty Crocker brownies lay in her path. She pushed it aside with her foot, and an old busybody scolded her for being too lazy to stoop over and pick it up.

"Someone else dropped it," my wife whispered to me, irritated, but too polite to confront her accuser.

"I'll take you in a wheelchair next time," I said. "Maybe people will leave you alone then."

The Department of Motor Vehicles issued us a handicap plate—length of time: indefinite. "I hope your wife feels better," the clerk in the office said kindly as she handed me the placard.

"I hope so, too."

Outside the supermarket, an old man stood with his hands on his hips. He watched me closely, frowning, as I parked the van in the handicap zone and exited the driver's side, a picture of health. Out of the corner of my eye, I saw an old woman up on the sidewalk doing much the same. Perhaps I should have faked a limp. I opened the back hatch and pulled out the wheelchair, and the old folks turned away, resuming their own lives.

I pushed my wife through the supermarket, while our daughter tried her best to keep up, pushing the shopping cart in something of a straight line, but occasionally careening off the soup cans.

As the cart grew heavy with groceries, our daughter's pace slackened until she could no longer make any headway.

"Here," I said, grabbing the front of the cart.

We made a train, my wife riding in front in her wheelchair, myself as the coupler between the wheelchair and the shopping cart, and our daughter, the caboose, steering the cart.

"Next time, you go shopping alone," my wife said softly as we rolled up to the cashier, more a spectacle than either of us cared to be.

Her doctor was no longer looking for a cure. He avoided words like 'terminal,' 'fatal,' 'incurable,' and opted for gentler terms—'unsatisfactory results,' 'runs its course.' He had hoped that the chemo—the low dose of 5-FU—would shrink the tumors and give her some relief from the pain. The tumors didn't shrink, but her blood counts did. Her hair disappeared, her blood disappeared, but the tumors remained. Then the mouth sores came.

"That's why they call it 5-FU," my wife said. "It's mostly F U."

Her blood counts collapsed even further.

"We may have to start transfusions," her doctor warned. He had started her up on Epogen—a blood builder—but he may have waited too long.

She lay in bed at night moaning. I adjusted her pillows, and her moans turned into whimpers.

"Just let me die," she whispered, her hoarse voice struggling against the mouth soars.

But I kissed her neck. "Please don't."

There was a shriek in the darkness; I sat upright in bed. Had I dreamt it? She shrieked again, and I knew it wasn't a dream, but our own nightmare. I turned on the small light that stood beside me on the night stand and looked over at her lying among the pillows, her eyes open wide, almost a look of terror. No, not terror—immense pain. I stared down at the pillows, and thought how easy it would be for me to pick one up and place it over her face, hold it there until her torment ended. No one would know—she'd been ill for so long. And even if they did find out, who would blame me?

I shook my head, angry at myself for even thinking such a thing. But I knew that it was the darkness, the screams, and not my own self that had conjured up such a thought. I knew that I could never hurt her.

Her eyes closed, and she slept again.

"I think we should increase the dose slightly," her doctor suggested. "Test the limits of your endurance."

She unbuckled the fanny pack and held it out toward him. "Enough," she said. "I'm ending it."

She caught both me and the doctor off-guard, but neither of us argued.

"It's your decision," he said uncertainly, looking to me for guidance.

"It's her decision," I agreed, a slight shrug of my shoulders, caught half-way between disappointment—disappointed that she would not fight on—and relief that her suffering would soon end.

"Maybe a little radiation, just to shrink the tumors and ease your pain," he suggested.

"Okay," she agreed. "A little radiation."

The radiation doctor frowned at her x-rays, zapped her for five days anyway, and the tumor in her upper spine disappeared. He smiled slightly, zapped her for five more days, and the tumor in her lower spine disappeared. He whistled old Disney tunes as he strutted from office to examination room, zapped my wife's hip seven times, and that tumor disappeared.

"It's really startling," her doctor observed. "We rarely see tumors react so quickly to radiation."

"I have a pain in my chest now," she said, cutting short his joy. "It's another tumor."

They did an x-ray, and she was right. She went back to the radiation doctor.

"Surprise. It's me again," she greeted him. "You should give me frequent fryer mileage."

He looked at her with a cool stare. "That's gallows humor," he replied. "We don't think that's funny here."

She repeated the joke to me that night when I got home from work.

"Don't you find that funny?" she asked. "I thought it was clever."

"I do, too," I answered. "I think if the patient can laugh at her predicament, then it's okay."

"Oh well," she sighed. "Other than his sense of humor, I like him."

"He probably sees too much suffering to find humor in his work," I suggested.

Chapter 29

❧

*I*T WAS LATE AUGUST.

"At least I'll get to see my daughter start school," she said sadly as she sat in her motorized armchair reading the local newspaper, checking the school bus routes. "Last year the bus stopped in front of our house." She ran her index finger down the list of addresses. "I don't see it."

From behind her, I scanned the list. "It stops next door this year," I noted, spotting the name of the nearest side street.

"That's good," she replied. "I can wheel myself to the window and see that she gets on safely then." She was in her wheelchair most of the time now—from weakness, not pain. The tumors were gone and the pain was gone, but so was her strength.

The following day, we received the official notice from the school informing us that our daughter was to walk to school.

"It must be a mistake," I suggested. "The school bus stops next door, but the school is half a mile away."

"That's a long way for a five-year-old to walk alone," my wife replied.

"There's an awful lot of turns, too," I agreed. "She'll never get there."

My wife sat glum in her armchair. "How do we get her to school now?"

"I'll take her in the first day. I'll take the day off from work," I decided. "I'll explain to the teacher that you're in a wheelchair and that the bus stops right next door."

"I suppose my mother can come over each day and bring her to school," my wife sighed. "Though I hate the idea of her getting in a car with my mother."

"Don't worry," I assured her. "They'll let her on the bus."

The first day of school arrived. The morning passed quickly for me and my wife, but passed slowly for our daughter. Too often she asked us what time it was, what time did school start, and how much longer she had to wait.

"Come on," I said. "We'll leave early. That way I'll have plenty of time to speak with your teacher."

My wife took our picture—we stood in the lawn, with roses in the background. She video-taped us as we walked together down the street toward the school, the two of us turning in unison, waving, as we reached the first corner.

We reached the second corner and I let my daughter take the lead, but she was already confused.

"It's just like going to the donut shop," I explained.

She hesitated, then turned the wrong way. My wife was right. There was no way she would show up at school if we sent her out the door on her own.

I met her teacher and explained that my wife had cancer and was in a wheelchair, that I worked in Boston so I was away during the day, and that the bus stopped next door. So can our daughter get on the bus, please?

She shook her head sadly. "You'll have to bring that up with the principal."

I found the principal whirling about in confusion. She managed to stop long enough to hear my story. "I'm sorry, but you live less than a half-mile from the school, so she can't take the bus," she instructed me, the tone of her voice suggesting that she thought I was one of her students. "That's the rule."

"The boy across the street takes the bus," I argued.

"He must be more than a half-mile from the school," she replied. I could see her eyes glancing over at a yardstick that hung beside her desk, yearning for something that measured precision—exactness—not something that could be argued with.

"But it's not safe for a little girl to walk that far by herself," I complained.

"She can't," the principal replied, frowning. "We won't let her leave here until a parent picks her up."

"Then this notice, where it says 'walker,' that's something of a fraud, isn't it?" I suggested. "You don't really expect her to walk."

"No, we don't." She smiled oddly, as if caught in a lie. "We expect the parents to provide them with transportation."

"But my wife's disabled, and I work in Boston," I said. "And the bus does stop right next door."

"I'm sorry," she said firmly. "I don't have any authority to assign buses. You'll have to call the superintendent's office." She wrote a phone number on a slip of paper, then snatched the paper up with her stubby fingers and handed it to me.

෴

"Did you straighten it out?" my wife asked. She had grown accustomed to me straightening things out, and did not expect that I would fail.

"No," I sighed.

She began to sob. "How could they be so cruel?" she asked plaintively. "It's just a little girl wanting to go to school."

"Don't cry," I said, stroking her stubbled hair. "I'll talk to the superintendent." I pulled the sheet of paper from my pants pocket and dialed the number.

No one picked the phone up at first. I began to wonder if they would pick the phone up at all. But then someone did, and said briskly, "yeah, hold," and I stood staring at my wife while I listened to a background of clattering old typewriters.

"You still there?" The woman returned, still brisk.

"Still here," I replied, then proceeded to tell her who I was, where I lived, and that I wished to put my daughter on the bus that stopped next door.

"We're not doing bus changes this week," she snapped. "Call back in two weeks."

I told her about my wife, about cancer and wheelchairs, about Boston and a small girl with a bad sense of direction.

"Look. We're busy. Write a letter," she growled. "We'll get back to you in two weeks."

"Two weeks?" I gasped. "Can I put her on the bus until then?"

"If you try to put her on the bus, she won't be allowed on," the woman shouted.

"How does she get to school?" I asked.

"That's your problem," the woman snapped, and hung up. It was the wrong thing for her to do.

I didn't need directions to the superintendent's office. I didn't know where it was—we were new in town—but I hunted it out as if the glow of toxic waste hung over the site. Paternal instincts.

I entered the outer office and dragged four years of shit in behind me, engulfing them so completely in a wake of unpleasantness that they didn't even ask who I was, but ushered me quickly into the superintendent's office so the rest of them could once again breath.

"We only have one rule," the superintendent explained patiently as he stood before an oversized map of the town, staring at a big red circle drawn around the kindergarten school building.

In the outer office, the clattering typewriters fell silent. The secretaries huddled together, listening, not sure what to do if gunfire erupted—run for their lives, or storm the superintendent's office with high heels flailing in a vain attempt to rescue a boss that none of them liked.

"If you live outside the half-mile radius, you can take the bus." He stabbed at the red circle with his chubby finger. "If you live inside, you can't." He folded his arms, certain that his presentation had been concise, accurate, and beyond dispute.

I found our house on the map. "But your line goes through our house," I pointed out. "Don't you think you can let her on the bus, considering the circumstances?"

"A half-mile is our only rule," he reiterated, tapping the red line.

"Is the bus full?" I asked, puzzled by his intransigence.

"Not at all," he replied flippantly. "But our only rule is a half-mile." He smiled, sure that I could understand such a neat and precise rule. "We'll send the safety officer out to measure it, just to make sure we didn't make a mistake."

"What about tomorrow?" I begged. "Can I put her on the bus until you decide?"

He glanced toward the door, along the bottom, and saw the

shadows of curious feet shuffling about on the other side. He lowered his voice. "Put her on," he whispered reluctantly, hating the sound of rules breaking. "But keep it under your hat, for me."

"They wouldn't let her on the bus?"

I shook my head.

"Crazy." My boss watched coffee pour into the empty pot. "They won't measure it, you know. I know bureaucracies. They'll say they measured it just to cover their asses, and say they were wrong, and you're further than a half-mile." He grew impatient and pulled the pot out from under the dripping water. A puddle formed on the counter.

"You think so?" I asked, waiting for him to fill his cup before holding mine out.

"Count on it," he said. "I know bureaucracies."

I called my wife, but she was already crying.

"I saw the policeman walk by our house," she sobbed. "He was pushing one of those measuring wheels."

"He was measuring?" I asked, shocked by what she told me.

"He pushed his little wheel right up to our front step." She cried again. "How could they be so cruel? She's just a little girl who wants to go to school. I'd take her if I could, but I just can't."

"Don't cry," I said. "She's getting on that bus."

The superintendent was expecting my call. Perhaps he knew we'd see the cop pacing outside our house with his little wheel.

"It's so heartbreaking," he explained. "So close. You're just twenty feet inside the circle."

I was about to reply with ugly threats of newspapers and reporters, but before I could say anything, he offered a solution. "For three hundred dollars, we allow children inside the circle to take the bus on an as-available basis."

"I see," I huffed. "Well, I'll put her on the bus then. You send us the bill, and I'll think about it."

They mailed us the bill, but I didn't send them a check. I sent them a letter instead, telling them how they made a sick woman cry on a day she had been looking forward to for years.

I never heard from them again after that.

Chapter 30

*S*HE WAS WALKING AGAIN, though lacking the energy she had the summer we hiked through Thomson Meadow. I attributed that—the energy loss—to the kindergarten incident.

"No," her doctor argued. "It's the radiation sapping her strength. We can't keep giving it to her." He had hope again, though. The tumors in her spine were gone, and so was the pain. When he saw her walk into his office under her own power, he smiled. "We can try tamoxifen again. That has no effect on the blood." He had found another tumor, a small one on one of her ribs. The radiation was working, but every time they killed one tumor, a new one grew. "It's like trying to even out the bumps in a rug," he explained. "We've got to try something systemic." He double-checked her record. "We haven't done hormone treatments in a few years."

"Okay," she relented. "But no more chemo. Ever."

We returned home, she lowered herself into her chair and closed her eyes.

"Are you okay?"

She opened her eyes slowly and smiled at me. "Take me to Hawaii."

"Hawaii?"

"Yes," she sighed. "We never went there together. We talked about it, but we never went."

"We have no money," I explained.

"None?"

"We have an equity credit line on the house," I said. "For emergencies."

"I'm not going to live through the winter," she replied, then slowly closed her eyes and swallowed.

This seemed to be an emergency.

The travel agent smiled blissfully as she calculated her commission in her head and thought of new shoes, that sharp-looking suit in the window of the department store, perhaps a membership at the health club all her friends belonged to.

"The Hyatt Regency in Maui, for ten days." I sat on the visitor's side of her desk and read aloud the carefully printed instructions my wife had given me.

"That's a great package." The woman smiled. "Anniversary?"

"More like a funeral," I replied, tearing a blank check from the credit line checkbook.

"I'm sorry," she said, but she saw the odd grin on my face and wondered whether there had been a joke that she had missed.

I scanned the next line of instructions. "There will be three of us. Two adults and a child."

"Would you like a rental car?" she asked, seeing me as a big bag of money, hoping for something extravagant—a bright red Mercedes convertible perhaps—so she could get a new scarf to go with that suit. But instead I asked for a mid-sized sedan, an odd bow to economy, and her smile faded slightly. She would have to get the scarf from her next client.

She clacked computer keys, pulling together hotels, planes, and cars, and frowned at her outdated green monitor. "Let's look over here," she said, not realizing "let's" means "let us," not "let me," keeping the screen hidden from my view.

"You're all set." She tore an itinerary from a noisy dot matrix printer and handed it to me. "You can come in next week for the boarding passes."

We sat together in the middle aisle holding hands. Her palms were sweating. Or was it my own sweat I felt? Takeoffs, landings—I hated them all now. We were a disaster area tearing through life, and all those who journeyed with us were in danger. Takeoffs were the worst—trying to go up, but then the plane deciding to go down. At least if we crashed during a landing, we were headed in the right direction.

Our daughter sat on my other side—glib, cheerful. An elderly woman grinned at her from the seat beside her.

The engines roared. My wife looked at me and smiled tensely. "What was that?"

"Flaps," I suggested.

"Oh. Flaps." She smiled again. She had felt the sweat, too. She wondered if it was hers or mine, but of course it was ours, sharing the same soul and sweating through the tense moments of life together.

Soon the plane would be off the ground. Already the wheels rattled free from the runway.

"What was that?" she asked, jumping slightly at the sound.

"Landing gear," I replied.

"Oh. The landing gear."

Soon we would be far away, removed from the earth, so far up we couldn't spit on it if we tried, evaporation taking its toll as the saliva tumbled further and further.

We had never told our daughter not to talk to strangers. At home, we told her to keep the rose bushes between her and strangers. She talked to everyone, sitting in her swing, pumping her legs, asking the mailman if he wanted to see how high she could go. Neighbors out walking their dogs stopped—and she'd tell them how she wanted to be an astronaut or maybe a dancer, and that her daddy didn't like it when their dogs peed on his roses.

How did we ever make her?

"Is this your first airplane ride?" The old woman grinned again at our daughter, unprepared for the response.

We should have hung a yellow caution sign around our daughter's neck—chatterbox on board.

"Oh no," our little traveler replied. "In June we flew to Aruba. I liked it there because it was hot and Dada took me to play miniature golf, but Mommy didn't really like it because it was windy, except she liked the restaurants and we ate goat, and the man on the boat spoke Portuguese which is a little like Spanish, which I'm trying to learn and I can count to ten already. Uno dos tres cuatro cinco seis siete ocho nueve diez. Before that, we flew to Florida. It always rains in Florida. I don't know why, but it does. My daddy says it's the family curse. We found sharks' teeth anyway."

We were passing over Kansas before she stopped for a breath of the dry cabin air.

I fell asleep and didn't wake until we crossed the Sierra Nevadas. I heard my daughter beside me.

"We didn't fly to Montreal, though. We drove and I skied with a French man, but he spoke English. I don't understand that. Why do they call him French?" She shrugged her little shoulders and the old woman laughed.

"I hope she didn't annoy you," I remarked.

"No, not at all," the old woman chuckled. "She had us all quite in stitches."

I looked around and saw the faces of our fellow travelers turned in their seats, smiling back at our daughter, and understood then why no one had rented the headphones.

"I'm sorry to have to leave you here, but I get off in San Francisco." The old woman touched our daughter's shoulder. "But you have fun in Hawaii."

The little girl sat still, oddly silent, so chatty yet never able to say good-bye.

My wife stirred beside me, kissing my neck. "She's a good little traveler, isn't she?" she asked, patting my hand.

I looked at her hand and noticed that the pasty color had disappeared, and was replaced by a rosy glow. Vacation therapy was working.

We were somewhere over the Pacific when our daughter finally asked, "When are we going to get there?" But by that time, I was asking myself the same question.

"Soon," I replied. "Take a nap."

"I'm not tired."

"When are we going to get there?" she repeated every few minutes.

"Take a nap," I suggested each time, but she wouldn't.

We were about to land when I realized she had been silent for some time. I looked over and saw that she had finally fallen asleep.

There was something wrong with Hawaii. We walked from our airplane through the open-air pavilion toward the luggage claim, palm trees on either side. Plumeria, bougainvillaea, orchids—it looked like Hawaii, but there was something not quite right. I looked toward my wife. She stared back with a tight, sad smile, and pulled her sweater tighter around her shoulders.

We talked of the volcano and whitecaps as we drove from the airport to the hotel, but said nothing of what we each had felt.

The bellboy opened the passenger door, stomping his feet and slapping his arms. He didn't greet us with the traditional Aloha, but instead stuttered out a convincing "cold."

My wife and I looked at each other—the family curse had followed us. "I thought it felt cold," she sighed.

"I thought so, too," I agreed. "But then I've never been to Maui."

"This usually only lasts a day or two," the bellboy remarked. Behind him, better prepared workers stood around wrapped in fall coats.

The bellboy was wrong, though. It didn't last only a day or two. Hawaii was hit by the worse stretch of weather since 1955. That was what the television weatherman said, and I believed him. For ten days the temperature hovered around seventy, not the customary eighty-two. The wind blew with such ferocity that the dive boats stayed tied up at shore for a week.

Palm trees bent half-way to the ground. The golfers finally surrendered, tired of seeing every shot they took blown into the Pacific Ocean. Instead, they spent their days learning new card games around the lobby of the hotel, stirring their drinks with little plastic golf clubs.

But despite the weather, the island had its effect—that mystical island ability to rejuvenate weary souls. My wife found she could stroll the streets of Lahaina and poke in the shops for souvenirs without fatigue. She stood in the shade of a banyan tree and admired the local art work, chatting cheerfully with the artists. We drove along the treacherous road to Hana and picnicked on the beach until the rain and the wind drove us to our car.

The wind let up a bit for a day, and we took a sailboat ride that followed the migrating whales. We watched them breach, huge, inspiring animals, so close to the boat that we felt we must be able to reach out and touch them. So close that I felt certain they were putting on a special show just to cheer her up.

We drove to the top of the volcano, breaking through the thick layer of clouds and into the cool sunshine above. We looked down across a billowy mass of white, so comfortable to look at—if only we could jump out far enough, the three of us, and land gently among them. So strange there above the clouds, like dwelling in the house of the gods. We had conquered Mount Olympus.

She feasted at the luaus, her appetite hearty again. I thought she might hula, but the native man passed her by and chose a younger woman.

I took my daughter snorkeling along the hotel beach where a wonderful reef came close to shore, and urged my wife to join us.

"You've got to come out and see the coral reef," I shouted. "It's quite beautiful."

She shook her head. "Too cold."

"The water's warm, though," I argued.

She shook her head again. "The air's still cold with the wind."

I drove us to Lahaina where the volcano sheltered the beach from the breeze. She eyed the rocks poking up through the water's surface.

"It's coral," I explained, trying to lure her into the water.

"Then the water's shallow?" she asked.

"Yes." I took her hand and led her to the water's edge.

She stepped nervously between the coral, along sandy paths formed randomly by nature's currents, meandering among the yellow brain coral, the graceful fan corals, and numerous other corals branching out more like trees than the animals that they were.

"Oh! Look at all the fish!" She bent low to the water, grabbing my arm for balance.

We were far from the hotels, along a stretch of beach known mostly to the locals, deserted now that it was a weekday. Rustic fishing huts lined the back of the beach, beyond the reach of the waves, shaded by an erratic row of palm trees.

"How did you find this place?" she asked. We sat together in the sand and watched our daughter as she collected shells in the shallows.

"I don't know," I shrugged. "I just knew it was here."

Then she joined our daughter and hunted for sea shells herself along the beach. Afterward, we drove toward the mountains and explored a protea garden. And that night, we dined beachside and watched the sun settle behind Molokai.

"I love you," she said to me as she watched the sunset, always finding more beauty in it than I ever did.

"I love you more," I replied, while our daughter smirked from behind a Shirley Temple, saying to herself, 'I love them like toast.'

The island magic—she was cured again. We had finally

traveled far enough, to a place where cancer would not come, to a speck of land at the center of a peaceful ocean. To where an agitated earth spit up its foul hot breath and created a paradise.

Chapter 31

✣

"YOUR TAN HAS FADED." Despite what he said, her doctor was obviously pleased by her appearance. "Any new pains?"

She shook her head.

"Any old pains?" he asked, and she shook her head again.

"She's even going to march in a parade this weekend," I boasted, wrapping my arms around her waist and giving her a little squeeze.

Her doctor raised his eyebrows in mocked surprise.

"With the kindergartners," she explained. "We'll only march part of the route."

"I'll be trailing behind them with a wagon," I remarked. "In case we have some stragglers." I grinned at my wife, letting her know that she could be a straggler if she wished.

"A parade." He examined her charts. "Well, why not. Your tumor marker's back to normal again, and your blood counts are near normal."

She stared at me in mild disbelief.

I answered her stare with a smile and a whispered word. "Snap."

We went to the parade route early and found the banner marking the meeting place for our daughter's school. My wife read the banner—class of 2008—then read it again, barely able to fathom a time so distant.

I stretched a thick rope along the sidewalk, marking the place where the children would wait. The plan was for them to sit patiently along the curb, to watch the parade for two hours, then hop in ahead of the local Junior High School band and march the last three blocks past the reviewing stand.

My wife had volunteered us to monitor eighty children. We were not alone, though. There were other mothers helping out—younger, presumably healthier mothers—serving punch on a day that was too hot for May, slathering sunscreen on the children's short white legs.

I watched my wife as she worked her way through the crowd of children. She avoided the younger mothers—they were a different generation of women, concerned with designer jeans and their European automobiles. Perhaps it wasn't a generation thing. Perhaps we had changed.

I steered unwelcome hordes of parade viewers away from the area, keeping strangers from mingling with the children. "Parade participants only," I announced, and endured the angry looks of the invaders as they walked away, staring longingly past the rope at the empty spots along the curb. "Sorry, there's more children coming." I waved my hands to keep them moving.

The mothers smiled appreciatively, glad for the few fathers that were helping out. Our masculine presence worked better against these interlopers than their motherly images would.

An aging group, saddled with too many lawn chairs and umbrellas, paused longer than most, seeming to object that children should get such a prime location. As I steered them away, an old man started spouting something about public sidewalks, and I started saying something about strangers among our children. A policeman wandered over and stood beside me, conveying to the group the official nature of what I was saying. They hefted their lawn chairs a bit higher and continued down the sidewalk, the man grumbling as he went, like an old Studebaker.

A mother spread blankets along the curb while I fought off the invaders. A teacher arrived and, with three words, ordered the children onto the blankets. I watched in amazement as the children went obediently toward the curb and sat down.

"Inside voices," the teacher commanded, and a hush fell over the children.

"It's great how well they behave," I said to my wife.

"It only lasts for a few years," my wife responded. "Then they aren't quite so respectful."

"And then they become teenagers," I said.

We both looked at one another—"Yuck!"—and laughed.

The parade began. Or rather, it arrived, for it had begun more than a mile away up Main Street. A clown danced by, taking one child by the hand and leading him into the street, not realizing that the child was part of a group. Seventy-nine children followed, fanning out like a chain of paper dolls. The clown stared back, surprised to find that the one child had multiplied into eighty. He led the children in a snake dance, then a conga line as a parade marshal scurried around in confusion, yelling, "you're too early! The children don't march until the third division!"

The teachers and the mothers stood on the edge of the curb watching, unsure of what to do, seeing that the children were having fun, but worried that the adults had ceded control to a clown. Then the clown turned back into the oncoming parade, weaving the children through a row of little carts driven by more clowns, and returned the children to the blankets.

The parade was too long and the children lost interest, scattering themselves among the trees of the nearby parsonage, finding shade and rest. Then a distant drumbeat called to us. The Junior High School band appeared on the horizon. We rounded up the children, gently shaking awake those who had fallen asleep in the cool shade.

The mothers lined up with the eighty children, my wife and my daughter standing side-by-side.

"I'm too old," my wife had sometimes complained. "I look like her grandmother," she'd say, and excuse herself from the school event. But there she was, not just under the scrutinizing eyes of the PTA, but for the whole town to see, standing tall and proclaiming Yes, I am old! Yes I may look like her grandmother, but I am her mother! I am the mother of the best little girl the world has ever seen, and I am the one that made her!

I marched at the rear, pulling the little red wagon, hearing the crowd applaud as we marched by, daydreaming that the applause was for my wife. The town officials, the guests of honor clapping wildly, beamed watermelon smiles at my wife. You've done it, and we love you for it! You are our hero!

I looked up into the reviewing stand and saw the quaint smiles directed at the youngest of the paraders—the class of 2008—and watched as the swarm of dignitaries turned their heads, drawn by the sour blast of trumpets, to greet the next contingent—the Junior High School Marching Band.

That night she sat rubbing her thigh.

"Did you trip or anything?" I asked.

She sat on the edge of the bed and rubbed higher. "I don't think so."

"Maybe you stepped in a pothole." I checked her leg under the reading lamp, but there were no bruises.

"No," she said. "You know what it is."

"But you're cured," I replied in a hushed tone.

Nothing. There is nothing there, she was told.

"There is something there," she argued. "There's pain there."

He looked more closely at the x-ray, standing so close to the view box that the image of bones reflected across his face. He hated this. Hard science said that she was fine, but he knew from experience that it was otherwise, that if she said there was something there, then there was.

Somehow she always knew, long before the tumor markers could measure it, well before the x-ray machines showed it as an indistinct blur.

"How do you know that's not a tumor?" I asked, pointing to a spot on the x-ray. "It looks different than the rest of the bone to me."

"They teach us to read these in medical school," he explained.

"Ah, I see," I replied. "Like reading tea leaves."

He smiled. "But I could be wrong. There could be a tumor there." He ordered a CAT scan.

The results came, and this time the test agreed with what my wife already knew—there was a tumor in her femur.

"You'll have to have more radiation," her doctor advised. "I'll call and set up an appointment."

"We're leaving for vacation on Wednesday," my wife replied.

"Again?" he asked in surprise. "To where?"

"Nova Scotia," I replied. "For a week."

"Well, we want to treat this pretty quickly," he explained. "We don't want the leg to break." He looked at my wife and examined the sadness in her eyes; he couldn't treat that. He knew her now. After five years of treatment, he felt that he knew her. "If I try to keep you here, you'll go to Nova Scotia anyway."

She nodded her head.

"Then we'll start your treatment once you get back." He picked up the phone to call the other doctor, the radiologist who didn't like gallows humor. "A one-week delay shouldn't matter that much," he said as he held his hand over the mouth piece and listened to the phone ring.

Chapter 32

WE DROVE FOR TWO DAYS before reaching the northern end of Nova Scotia and the island of Cape Breton. In the town of Baddeck, a village lined with Scottish inns, the sun shone briefly on Bras d'Or Lake, luring us to an inn on the shoreline that sat nestled among the pines.

My wife had asked me to get a room downstairs, but in the confusion of checking in, it slipped my mind. We stood together at the bottom of the long staircase, looking up.

"I could go ask for another room," I offered.

"It's okay," she sighed. "My leg doesn't hurt that much."

"They have more rooms," I said. "It's Sunday. Everyone's checking out."

"No," she stated firmly. "I'll be fine." She grabbed the banister and climbed slowly to the landing where, to her relief, she spotted our room number on a nearby door.

"I could get us another room," I repeated, but she shook her head slowly.

"I'll be fine."

We dined that night in a slopeside restaurant with a view of the lake. While we ate, a Scotsman sat on a small stage and sang folk songs from his native land, and winked at our daughter between songs, calling her a fine young lass. It was a buffet, so we felt obliged to overeat. And afterward, we walked the excess off along the shoreline. Our daughter caught crabs beside a small dock and announced that the lake was salty.

"Don't drink from the lake!" My wife frowned at the little girl and shook her head slowly in disbelief.

"But it's salty!"

Briny, someone told us, not salty. Not quite an ocean, and not quite a lake.

"Then we don't need a fishing license?" I asked, thinking we could drop a line in without too much hassle. But we did need a license. Salt water fishing didn't require a license, but briny water fishing did.

On the east coast of the island sat the restoration of Fortress Louisbourg, a French stronghold sacked by the British in the early years of the European conquest. Dark clouds threatened rain, but we drove toward the ancient town anyway, knowing that the sun would not shine that day, but hoping that the rain would not fall either. A tour bus drove us from the visitor center to the edge of the town, where we disembarked before a reconstruction of the original town gates.

"It's too far to walk," my wife cried, looking past the two colonial soldiers to the town itself.

"They said there were wheelchairs available." I looked about, but there was only a fisherman's hut nearby. I opened its door and peered in, catching the family by surprise as they sat around a rude table in the light of a candle. But they were not real fishermen—they were actors and actresses dressed in period clothes, there to portray the life of a colonial fisherman's family.

"Do you have a wheelchair?" I asked.

A woman went into a back room and returned dragging one out. She invited us to come in, to watch them as they went about their daily chores, but we declined and rolled on toward the walls of the town, as all the other visitors had done.

"We should have gone in," I reflected.

"Why?" my wife asked.

"I don't know. They seemed lonely."

The rain started to fall, and the wheels of the wheelchair began to sink into the mud. We sought shelter in one of the exhibits, but could not get the wheelchair over the doorjamb.

"I can walk," she said, and got up hurriedly, losing her footing on the slick surface of the mud.

I grabbed her arm before she fell. "In here," I said, and steered her toward a different door, into an old-time inn with wooden benches and communal tables.

"That's better," she sighed as we entered a dry alcove. I pulled her dripping raincoat from her shoulders.

We shared a table with two other couples—a husband and wife from Ontario, and a man and a woman. The man and the woman were not a couple, but hikers or campers who had come together in some peculiar way that I could not quite figure out.

The storm eased up just enough to coax us onto the streets again, but then the rain began to fall in sheets.

"Let's go back to the visitor's center," my wife suggested. "There's a gift shop there."

"Shopping, yes!" our daughter shouted, the only words she

had spoken since the guard at the town gate had asked her "who goes there?"

The next day, we left Baddeck and the briny waters of Bras d'Or Lake, driving past our second bald eagle of the trip, sitting boldly in the branches of a dead tree. We drove along the east coast through an area the guide book described as a plethora of quaint villages and rugged coastline, but the heavy fog prevented us from seeing more than an occasional steeple and the casualties of the night before—porcupines splattered across the road. The clouds broke apart as we approached Halifax, and we entered the suburbs under brilliant sunshine.

Halifax itself was a modern city, busy, yet quiet. Clean and unhurried.

"They have a casino," my wife noted, pointing to the marquee over our hotel.

"The guide book doesn't mention it," I replied. "Maybe it's not a gambling casino."

"What kind of casino would it be?" she asked.

"I don't know. Like at Newport, where they have a casino but play tennis or something there."

"It is gambling casino," the doorman agreed. "It just open." He was a pleasant man from Nigeria who had arrived in New York but continued on to Halifax, finding the racial climate there much better—the English and French were too busy fighting over language to worry too much about skin color. "You leave car here. Go check in hotel."

"Did you lock the car door?" my wife asked me.

The pleasant man from Nigeria just laughed. "You don't worry about that here," he said. "Nobody steal car."

I shrugged and walked toward my wife.

"Humor me," she said. "I'll feel better if it's locked."

The doorman smiled. "You do what wife say. That always best. But I tell you, nobody steal car here."

I tipped him five, then realized it was Canadian, and tipped him another five. He smiled broadly. "You leave car here and don't worry."

We didn't unpack, but went straight out for a stroll, glad for the sunshine. Rush hour approached, and the streets were busy as we neared the first crosswalk.

"Did you see that?" I said, shocked. "They stopped."

"They're supposed to stop," my wife replied. "We're in a crosswalk."

"But they stopped before we even got to the crosswalk." I waved to the patient motorists and they waved back.

"You've been working in Boston too long," she laughed.

We visited the waterfront, an area friends had told us to avoid, an area they had described as a collection of seedy bars, drunken sailors, and prostitutes. But we found it had been restored, or perhaps reinvented, and was now a pleasant pedestrian mall lined with shops and fine restaurants.

We stopped at a shop that specialized in native crafts, where my wife bought a hand-made cane and my daughter bought a stuffed animal fashioned from the pelt of a seal.

We exited the shop and stepped into the evening sun.

"Let's eat," my wife suggested.

"How about there." I pointed to an upstairs cafe with a seafaring name.

"Seafood sounds good," she said.

"What about the stairs?"

"I can make it." With the help of her new cane and the banister, she made it to the top, only to find out they had an elevator in back for the handicapped. I rewarded her efforts with a frozen Margarita.

After dinner, we stopped at a nearby tent that protected a series of touch tanks—a nautical petting zoo of sorts—where my daughter squealed in delight as she pulled a sea cucumber out of the tank and it squirted sea water all over her blouse.

One tank held sting rays. We felt their velvety skin as they swam past us, gliding silently by over and over again until I wasn't sure if we were petting their backs or they were petting our fingers.

"I'm getting tired," my wife sighed. "Let's head back to the room."

We returned to the hotel, my wife tapping her new cane against the cobblestones as we went.

Halifax sprawled before us in the morning light, built upon a hill that overlooked the busy harbor. We stood outside our hotel, at the bottom of the steep hill, and looked up toward the citadel—our goal.

"Let me get the van," I offered.

"I can make it," she replied stubbornly.

I studied the tourist guide for a moment, then pointed to a glass structure nearby. "That's the pedestrian mall. It'll get us partway up the hill."

We took the pedestrian mall as far as we could, then continued toward the citadel by entering buildings on the downhill side, taking their elevators up a flight or two, and exiting on the uphill side. A man noticed our maneuvers and offered his help.

"Follow me," he said. "I'll show you the best way up that hill."

We were leery as we followed him through a deserted hallway and into an empty elevator. We rode up in silence. The elevator opened and we found ourselves on the sidewalk at the base of the citadel.

"How was that?" he asked.

"Great," I replied. "Thanks."

There was not another elevator, though. From the base of the citadel, a staircase led up the grassy slopes, past the white clock tower, and up to the fortress. My wife decided to wait below.

"I can go back and get the van," I offered again. "There's a road that goes up there."

"No," she said, setting herself on a bench. "I've seen enough forts."

Our daughter went ahead of me, counting each of the wooden steps as she climbed.

"You're skipping some," I said.

"No I'm not," she argued, then counted, "thirty-two, thirty-three," saying nothing as she stepped onto a wide landing, then continuing, "thirty-four," as she stepped from the landing to the tread above.

"The wide one's a step, too."

She continued climbing—"forty-eight forty-nine"—and stepped toward the next landing.

"Fifty," I said as her toe touched down, but she covered her ears and scooted across the landing, calling out a very distinct fifty of her own as she hopped up onto the step above.

We reached the last step and decided to stop there. "I've seen enough forts, too," I said.

"Yeah," she agreed. "We've seen enough."

We ran down the staircase, she counting the steps and I counting the landings. Out of breath, we ran to where my wife sat.

"A hundred and twenty-two steps," the little girl yelled.

"A hundred and forty-two," I corrected her. "She skipped the landings."

"Okay," my wife sighed. "At least you had fun."

"There's handicap parking at the top," I informed her. "I could get the van and drive you up."

"No. That's okay." She studied the tourist map briefly, then pointed to the left of the citadel. "The Public Gardens are over that way. Could we see them?"

"Sure." I took my wife's hand and helped her from her seat. "You want me to get the van?"

"No, I can walk," she assured me.

Her happiness grew, and each step lightened as we entered the gates to the garden. She was a hummingbird set free among the nectar, her wings clipped, unable to flit from blossom to blossom, but pleased by the promise of a bountiful future. She sat on a concrete bench and pointed to individual flowers with her cane, naming them as though they were lost friends.

"Forsythia. Honeysuckle. Ageratum. Tulips. Dianthus. Sweet William."

I pointed to a yellow border. "Daffodils."

"No. Narcissus," she corrected me.

"I can never keep those two straight," I replied.

She rose slowly from the bench and walked into a bed of tea roses.

"Do they make tea out of them?" our daughter asked.

We went as far as the fountain and sat watching as children played, sticking their fingers into the falling water. A throng of retirees—a tour group from North Carolina—flooded the area with their matching red T-shirts and khaki pants, their uniformity seeming ugly and distracting despite their flower bed appearance.

She frowned. "I'm tired," she sighed. "Let's go back to the hotel."

That night she lay on our bed, moaning slightly as she rubbed her leg. "I shouldn't have done so much walking."

The television played in the background. They were warning of an approaching hurricane, but we had seen the news flash already and ignored it as they repeated the report for their late viewers.

"You'll rest tomorrow," I said. "We'll go for a drive. Then Saturday we'll get up early and take the ferry home."

"We can't take the ferry," she sighed. "There's a hurricane coming."

"I called. They said the ferry would still run in a hurricane."

"It can run without us," she said firmly.

We watched the weather closely. Throughout the following day, we listened to the reports on the car radio as the hurricane made a beeline for us, promising to cross the Gulf of Maine at the same time we would.

The family curse.

But looking about as we drove through the countryside, there was no evidence of a storm. The sun shone brightly. We parked and looked out across the beaches—huge caverns scooped out by the surging tides of the Bay of Fundy, the cliffs of shale and clay collapsing into piles among the sand like giant elephant droppings.

A rough dirt road led us through a farmer's desolate fields and deposited us in a rustic parking lot. Two other cars sat among the weeds.

"See?" I said. "We weren't the only ones to come here." In the distance, we saw a lighthouse. We climbed the narrow stairs and stood looking over the railing at the pounding surf below, the brown waters of the Fundy, the tide—a spectacle—invading the nearby cove, racing across the broad expanse of sand until the beach was gone.

She leaned over the railing, her thoughts joined with mine. It would be so easy. Just lean over, keep leaning, lean until the world was upside down, then drop softly into the sea, and it would all be over.

But remember your daughter. I sent the message along the invisible thread that had connected us all our lives. It reached her, entered her through her cheek like a kiss, and she turned and smiled.

And you, her smile said, I could never leave you, either.

⌘

We boarded the ferry despite the approaching hurricane. She was tired, and to drive around the Bay of Fundy and through New Brunswick would be too tedious. The boat ride was tedious, though. Eight hours through fog and heavy seas.

"It's not as rough as I thought," she remarked, almost disappointed that the hurricane wasn't more of a storm, something to add a little excitement to an uneventful cruise.

I took our daughter to the slot machines. She quickly learned the technique, dropping a coin and pulling the arm down with the speed of a seasoned pro. Strobe lights blinked and bells rang, creating excitement for the little girl. Two women stood behind us, whispering. I knew what they were saying—such an evil man, teaching a young girl to gamble— but I didn't care. Our life was different than theirs. The perils we saw were much larger than the loss of a few quarters.

My intent was for her to lose her money, to use our experience together as an opportunity, a chance to teach her the folly of gambling. But she kept winning. Quarters fell from the machine and filled her cup to overflowing.

She ran back to the small parlor where her mother sat. "See how much I won!"

My wife stared over at me. "You let her gamble?"

"She was supposed to lose," I shrugged. "I was trying to teach her something about gambling."

The little girl poured some of her coins into her mother's lap, making room in the cup for more winnings. "Come on, Dada." She grabbed my hand and dragged me toward the slot machines. "Let's play some more."

The second time was not so kind. The quarters disappeared until a half-dozen were left scattered in the bottom of her cup.

"You're still ahead," I pointed out.

"Let's stop," she decided. "Let's go to the gift shop and spend these."

She had learned a valuable lesson after all—when to quit.

"This is like the hospital," my wife complained. We had moved to one of the boat's lounges and sat hunched over a low coffee table. Cards and a cribbage board were scattered across the surface. "How much longer?"

I looked at my watch. "An hour."

"Next time we drive," she sighed.

"We did it backwards," I observed. "I think what you want to do is take the ferry to Nova Scotia. That's a night crossing and you can sleep through it. Then you drive home."

The ferry had been blowing its lonely fog horn throughout the journey, but now we were hearing distant replies and knew that we were approaching the coast of Maine. The other passengers started gathering up their possessions, also knowing that the trip was near its end.

The public address system crackled with customs instructions.

"We'd better get to the elevator," my wife suggested.

A large crowd had already formed in front of the elevator door. My wife scanned the crowd. "We'll take the stairs."

It was a wide curving staircase, carpeted in a deep red to give it an air of opulence. She took one step, then suddenly sat down, dropping her cane through the banister and onto the heads of the people below.

I looked down at her face and saw the stark whiteness of her skin. "What's wrong?"

"My leg broke," she whispered.

A woman stopped to help. She took my wife's arm, wanting to lift her, but my wife shook her head. "Don't," she cried. "My leg's broken."

Other passengers hurried past. She had not fallen, but had merely sat down—she couldn't be hurt, could she? Even I doubted what she said.

The woman pressed down on her shoulders. "Don't move. I'll get some help."

She returned quickly with a man in a uniform. The two stooped beside her. "Can you get up?" the man asked.

"I have a tumor in my leg," she replied, "and the bone just broke."

A crowd gathered, unsure of what help they could offer. I stood among them, but remained isolated by the feeling that we had entered a nightmare in which others did not belong. Our daughter huddled under my arm, hiding in silence. "She has breast cancer," I said, feeling the odd nature of the accident needed further explanation.

The paramedics arrived and pushed the first woman aside. She could offer no further help, but she wanted to remain, to offer her support to the small family. She picked up a stuffed animal and handed it toward our daughter.

"Here," she said softly. "A little girl left it on the steps for you." As she placed the furry red lobster in our daughter's arms, the woman reached out and stroked her hair.

My wife sat with her lower leg bent under her good leg, unmoved since the accident. The woman paramedic felt along the length of the bent leg. "I don't think it's broken," she said. "I think you got a cramp."

She tried to pull the leg straight, but my wife responded with a scream of agony. The scream reached my ears and my daughter's ears like an unexpected volley of arrows. My daughter covered one ear with her palm and started screaming, too, pressing the toy lobster harder and harder against

230

her other ear until its eyes bugged out. The crowd that had gathered spun away from the cries—it was no longer a spectacle, but a session of torture that they could no longer endure. The first woman still lingered, though. She placed her hand on my shoulder and led me through the silent crowd toward the stairs, nodding toward my daughter. "Perhaps you should take her someplace quiet," she instructed. "I'll stay with your wife."

I went reluctantly, feeling that I was abandoning my wife to strangers who could not possibly understand what she felt. But I knew it was best for the child. To leave her standing there while her mother screamed, with her screaming in unison. . . No, it was best for me that we left before I started screaming, too.

"Why don't I faint," my wife hissed through clenched teeth. She looked up at me, the pain glowing moist in her eyes as I stepped carefully past her. "You're supposed to faint when the pain is this bad."

"You're too strong." I leaned over and kissed her gently, afraid that the touch of my lips would break another part of her. "You've always been strong, and now it's working against you."

I clutched my daughter as she clutched her lobster, and together, reluctantly, we climbed down the curved staircase and left the ferry boat.

I pushed two chairs together, making a small bed in the lobby of the hospital. A nurse watched over my sleeping daughter as I went to the van and dug through the luggage for our beach towels. I returned with the towels and spread them over my daughter.

"Thank you," I said to the nurse.

"My pleasure," she replied, pausing briefly to take one last look at the peaceful child before returning to the chaos of the emergency room.

Two children with a baby paced the lobby. They might have been sixteen, but no older. The girl's teeth were black with decay. When the boy talked, his blank stare and his pronounced overbite conspired to give him the appearance of a ventriloquist's dummy.

"Why don't they take us," the boy complained. "That other man, his head's just bleeding, but our baby got green stuff coming out of hers." He wiped the green snots from the baby's face with his sleeve.

The girl took the baby from the young father's arms, cooing, "baby be all right, baby be fine," like they had never gotten around to giving their offspring a proper name.

The hospital staff had yet to tell me anything about my wife—whether the leg was broken, even. I had gone to the front desk to register, but the woman there told me to take a seat, that she would be with me shortly. I had waited long enough and I needed to find my wife. But I needed someone to watch my daughter while I was gone. I spotted a woman in the corner who 'fell down the stairs.' Beaten by her husband was more likely. A drunk paced the floor, swearing that he was having a heart attack and no one would listen to him.

A stretcher rolled past with a girl having a seizure, a drug overdose. Her parents sat down beside me, the mother crying, her hands folded—writhing—in her husband's lap. Would I entrust my daughter to strangers who had failed with their own child?

Two women entered and sat down behind me, well dressed, mother and daughter. The younger one was pregnant but of a proper age and wearing a ring.

"Could you watch my daughter for a few minutes?" I asked.

They smiled pleasantly. "Of course."

I went to the nurse's station and found out where they were holding my wife. Her voice reached me in the hallway, tense, aggravated. I entered her room and found her lying on a gurney, the woman from the front desk hovering over her asking her questions about insurance coverage. I took the woman's arm and pulled her away. "I'll tell you what you need to know," I hissed, and pointed to the hallway. "Sit down and I'll be with you in a few minutes."

My wife smiled upon hearing my voice. "Hi, honey."

I went over and touched her shoulder. "Is it broken?"

"They haven't x-rayed yet," she sighed. "The doctor thinks so, though."

"You've been here over an hour," I complained. "What have they been doing?"

"They were trying to get insurance information before you chased that woman away."

"That's all?"

She nodded slowly, then began to cry. "I've ruined everything again."

"The vacation was over with anyway." I began rubbing her shoulder with my fingertips, up toward her neck where I knew she liked it most. "It's just a broken leg. They can fix that."

The doctor entered. "We have to take her to x-ray now."

I kissed her gently.

She looked around, frantic, like a trapped animal, understanding for the first time that our daughter was not with me. "What did you do with her?"

"Relax," I purred. "She's sleeping in the lobby. Two women are watching her."

"You left her with strangers?"

"What else could I do?" I replied. "Besides, they looked okay."

She tried to raise herself from the gurney, but I pushed her down with a gentle palm. "Relax."

Relax. There was nothing more to do. The cards were dealt, our fateful hand was drawn. It was only in how we played the game that the outcome could be changed.

Chapter 33

❧

"**T**HE SURGEON said my wife would be in her room by one o'clock." I held my watch up for emphasis, and turned it toward the nurse. "It's now five o'clock."

She shrugged her shoulders. "All I can tell you is that your wife is fine."

"Except she's still in recovery," I said angrily, "and not in her room."

The nurse shrugged again.

I had driven home through the night, dropped our sleeping daughter off at my sister-in-law's, driven to our house for a short nap, called my wife's doctor to inform him of the situation, phoned the surgeon in Maine—the one who was going to put my wife's leg back together—then jumped in the van and hurried back to Maine so I could be there when my wife woke up from the anesthesia.

Now I was cranky.

I paced in front of the nurses' station until my anxiety rubbed off onto the entire staff, then I returned to the little waiting room and sat watching the housekeepers as they snuck onto the balcony for forbidden cigarettes. The women, their mops abandoned by the doorway, spoke Russian amongst themselves while the little Puerto Rican man stood silent, leaning on his broom, smiling to himself as he watched their large rumps.

Finally, a gurney rolled down the hall. A nurse poked her head into the waiting room, frowned for a moment at the women smoking on the balcony, then signaled for me to follow her.

I sat down beside my wife and whispered in her ear. "It's me, honey."

"Uh." She opened her eyes until the daylight shut them again. "Uh."

"Don't talk," I whispered.

She didn't.

"Don't worry about anything," I said. "Your sisters have moved into action on the home front." I knew that would make her happy. Her sisters were very efficient, natural-born planners.

She tried to say our daughter's name.

"She's staying with your sister," I replied softly. "I won't bring her here. She'll visit you once you're back in Boston."

I explained to her what I knew, what her treatment would be. A few days in the hospital, then a few weeks at a nursing facility for physical therapy. She seemed to be asleep as I prattled on and on, except for the few times she swallowed hard.

Then I was silent as I sat staring at her face, trying to

remember the last time I had seen her smile without an edge of sadness to it. The shadows of the evening fell through the window, rousing me from my thoughts. I kissed her sleeping cheek and went home.

The insurance company had abandoned Kalamazoo; my onslaught had been too intense for them. They had retreated south to the border to regroup. Monday morning, I was talking to one of their clerks in Texas.

"I'm sorry," she said, her twangy southern accent hurting my ear. "Your policy doesn't pay for transportation."

"We're not talking about a cab ride," I argued. "She needs an ambulance. Her doctor wants her transferred to Boston so he can oversee her treatment."

"That's transportation," she replied.

"Let me explain." I shifted my grip on the phone receiver as if preparing for a tug-of-war. "She's in intensive care right now. If you transfer her to Boston, she'll be in a nursing facility, which is a lot cheaper. You'll save money in the long run."

"We'll send her to a nursing facility, if that's what you want," the Texan explained. "But we'll choose where she goes, and we can send her farther away from you if we choose to."

I was beginning to feel glad for the Alamo. "Then I won't authorize her release, and you can keep paying for intensive care."

Humph. I hung up the phone with enough force to rattle her teeth.

The social worker at the Boston nursing facility got involved. "We'll hold her bed for a week," she explained. "I should be able to get her transferred by then."

"How much will it cost if I have to hire an ambulance?"

"Thousands," she said.

"Thousands?"

She nodded solemnly. "But don't worry. We'll work something out."

I went to work early each morning, then caught the afternoon train home, changed my clothes, and drove to Maine to visit my wife for an hour or so.

"When are you taking me home?" she asked sadly.

"Soon," I promised, then kissed her good-bye and drove to my sister-in-law's, stopping along the highway for a fish sandwich.

They were finishing dinner when I arrived. We sat at the kitchen table and watched my daughter roll peas around her dinner plate. It was Thursday now. My wife still languished in a Maine intensive care unit, a pawn in an insane battle between me and the insurance company, the dollars flowing by faster and faster, far surpassing the cost of an ambulance ride.

Don't give in, she had told me, and I didn't.

My daughter rose from her seat. She walked shyly to my side and hugged my waistline. I looked down and saw tears under her long black eyelashes. "What is it, Sweetie?" I asked.

"I want to go home." She began to sob, and I pulled her to my lap and hugged her. "I just want to go home with you. Can't I?"

"Of course you can, Pumpkin." I kissed her forehead, then her cheek. She threw her arms around my neck and squeezed hard enough to choke a smaller man. "I thought you were having fun here with all your cousins."

She shook her head. "I want to be with you."

I stood up, the little girl hanging from my neck, and smiled meekly at my daughter's hosts. "I'm sorry."

But they waved away my apology. "Don't be silly. We understand." They gathered her things and carried them to the van as I walked out with my daughter still clinging desperately to my neck.

We stopped at a restaurant for dessert, father and daughter. She looked at me from across the table and smiled as she sipped a root beer float through a straw. Then a sadness flooded her face, and she said with more courage than I would ever have expected, "I guess from now on, it's just you and me, Dada."

No, I whispered to myself. Your mother will live to be a hundred.

There was a message on the answering machine when we got home. The insurance company had surrendered and my wife would be coming home the next day. Not home home, but to Boston to the nursing facility. It would feel like a homecoming, though.

She showed me all her new toys—objects designed to help the immobile: a plastic sock holder with two ropes so she could pull her socks on by herself; a personal potty seat so she wouldn't have to travel so far—extra high so she wouldn't have to squat.

"What's that?" I pointed to an odd object on her table.

She picked it up—a type of gripper with a string mechanism—and pulled its trigger, pinching my nose. "That's my claw. So I can pick things off the floor."

"You never picked things off the floor before," I teased.

"Watch it buster, or I'll pinch your butt," she laughed, pulling the trigger three times, clamping the claw in the air. She set the gripper aside. "I started physical therapy today."

"That's good," I observed. "What about radiation?"

"I'll start that next week." She stared out the window, and I could read her thoughts—summer again, another summer in the hospital.

I returned from a meeting and saw the red light flashing on my office phone. I pressed the playback button and listened. The message was hurried, somewhat garbled. "The doctor . . . the leg . . . they're going to operate . . . I need you." Then she broke down in tears.

I ran to the elevator, my mind racing. What had she meant? There had been a lot of damage from the tumor, the bone eroded away then snapped in two, now held together by a rod shoved up the center of each half of a shattered femur. Then it struck me. They were going to amputate. I turned away from the subway entrance and headed instead to the taxi stand, needing the speed of a private vehicle to get me to my wife's side before they inflicted more pain on her.

I raced up the hospital stairs two at a time, then rushed through the secret passages of the lower level, using the short cuts I had discovered over the years. Through the kitchen area, the cooks pausing to look, wondering if I was another state inspector. Through unmarked doors and nameless hallways until I emerged before the desk of the nursing facility.

"Hello," a nurse called as I brushed past and hurried to my wife's room.

I found her lying there like a stone, the television on, but her eyes staring off toward a meaningless corner of the room.

"I got here as fast as I could," I gasped, sitting down on the edge of her bed and taking her in my arms. "What's wrong?"

She pointed to a crude pencil drawing, a picture of a broken leg.

"That's what your leg looked like?" I asked.

She shook her head. "That's what it looks like now."

I pulled the picture closer to my face. "It still looks broken."

She nodded. "The doctor in Maine didn't do the procedure correctly." She sobbed gently as she spoke. "She didn't believe you when you told her I had a tumor, so she treated it like a regular fracture." She took the drawing from my hand. "It broke again."

"What are they going to do now?" I waited to hear the 'A' word. Am . . . am . . . am . . . am . . . ampu. . . .

"They want to do it correctly," she cried. "They need to put some plates or something on the bones. I'll have to go back to ICU for a week, and then start physical therapy all over again."

I held her close, relieved. "But at least they aren't amputating your leg."

"Oh, I wish they would," she cried. "I don't need it. I'm never getting out of here, anyway."

It was August when she finally left the hospital. An entire month lost. We waited impatiently for the orderly to arrive and wheel her out. I offered to fetch her wheelchair from the van and dash her away myself, but my wife had no wish to upset their procedures.

"To hell with their procedures," I snapped. "What are they going to do? Have us arrested?"

"Shush," she said. "We waited this long. We can wait a few minutes more."

They had not finished her radiation treatments, so for

two weeks afterward, we returned each day to Boston for her session.

"Why didn't they do it while they had you in the hospital?" I asked angrily.

She shook her head, unsure of why they did anything the way they did at this point. "You won't get in trouble leaving work early?"

"I go in early," I explained.

"It's just I like it when you drive me."

That was difficult to believe, recalling our daily journeys into Boston, her little shrieks as cars zipped past us on the right, her constant warnings about lunatics coming up fast on the left. But I knew they were responses to others, not an indictment of my own driving skills. She feared the world now. Her peace had been long-since shattered.

My mother-in-law came each day to watch our daughter and to help around the house. I had invited her to move in when the leg first broke, but she remembered how our daughter had reacted two years before when she stayed with us during the bone marrow treatment. Grandmother and granddaughter were pals now, and she didn't want to upset that.

"It's not getting any better," my wife moaned. The physical therapist had just left. She had been doing physical therapy, but then they stopped it, wanting to give her leg a chance to heal. Now her surgeon had started it up again.

Her doctor switched her to Arimidex, another hormone therapy. The tamoxifen had done its job, keeping the cancer at bay for six months. But cancer was crafty. It had discovered that it was being duped into eating the deadly tamoxifen and refused offers of more. So her doctor tried another hormone,

one the cancer hadn't seen yet, hoping that perhaps he could trick it again. For another six months, anyway.

"What happens after that?" my wife asked anxiously.

"There's another hormone," her doctor answered. "A male hormone. Women don't like the side effects much."

"Like facial hair and a deeper voice?" she asked.

He shook his head. "Nothing like that."

She shook the suggestion off anyway. "Never mind. I'll stick with Arimidex."

She could no longer climb the stairs each night. She tried the first two nights, struggling up each step, using a crutch and the banister for support, but the effort was too much.

"It was that second operation," she sighed. "Too much trauma."

"I'll move the guest bed into the parlor for you," I offered. "I could sleep there, too. If you want."

"No. The bed's too small," she replied. "Besides, you kicked my leg last night."

"I'm sorry," I said. "I didn't mean to."

"No," she sighed. "You didn't mean to, but you did."

I kissed her goodnight each evening, leaning over her as she lay sideways in the bed, the only position that seemed comfortable for her anymore. My lips searched under the covers for hers, our two lips meeting, touching. A brief touch. "Good night."

"Good night," she replied.

I lingered for a moment, thinking there must have been more I could do. "Sleep tight."

"Good night," she replied.

Lingering a bit longer, feeling a hollowness growing, I'd whisper, "Don't let the bed bugs bite."

≈

"Why don't you leave me?" she asked.

She had heard me climb the stairs from the basement, carrying up the last load of clean laundry. I set the basket down beside her motorized recliner and started sorting and folding towels.

"It would be so easy," she declared. "Get a divorce, marry someone else, someone who's not defective like me. You'd have a life again."

"I could never do that." I gave the towel more critical attention than I did her suggestion. How many years ago had she told me to throw that one out? It was still with us. And I was still with her, both of us as ragged as the towel, perhaps.

"Why haven't you left me?" It was not idle chatter. Her voiced begged for an answer.

I placed the folded towel on a snack table and thought for a moment. Why hadn't I left her? Because her sisters would kill me? Because our daughter would suffer? Because I loved her, and promised to love her through sickness and in health? It was many of these things. All of them. Commitment, love, fear, sometimes pity. And sometimes it was none of them at all, but sheer habit that kept me there. But I couldn't explain it fully to myself and to try explaining it to her would only make her cry.

"Because I'm selfish," I suggested, and yanked another tattered towel from the laundry basket.

"Selfish?" She laughed. "You have no life anymore. How could you be selfish?"

"Because people know I have no life," I explained. "They look at me, and admire me for what I'm doing. I'm selfish and greedy and thrive on the admiration."

"Only a few people even know I'm sick," she argued. "How much can that be worth?"

"Enough that I stay here with you," I replied.

She looked at me and knew I was joking, that I didn't really care what anyone thought of her or me. I thought she would smile, finding humor in my damaged view of the world, but she didn't.

"You never should have married me," she stated, then exhaled as though the effort of speaking had exhausted her.

But then our daughter entered, joyful, holding up the drawing she had just made, wanting to show it off, and we both knew that my wife was wrong.

Perhaps I should have married her earlier.

We clapped our hands as the little girl spun about with the drawing held high over her head.

She bowed, then turned to leave. "I'm going to make Mommy a get well card next!" she announced, happy with the success of her artistic endeavor.

"I'm never getting well," my wife said once our daughter was gone, standing for a moment, the only exercise she could now do. She would take a few steps to the kitchen counter, turn, then come back. She called it her daily walk.

"Of course you are," I replied, and set the last piece of laundry aside. "The bone is already healed."

"But I'm not healed," she groaned. "I've been broken too many years."

I reached out and pulled her toward me. "Then I'll be your glue." I squeezed her to my chest. "I'll hold you together."

"What will you do when I'm gone?"

Go on, I thought. What more? Just go on. Drift through the fog, try to find my way. But I didn't say that. What I said was, "You'll live to be a hundred."

She smiled sadly. "Take care of our daughter," she begged, looking longingly toward the dining room where the little girl sat with her crayons and her sheets of construction paper, scraps of pink and yellow fluttering to the ground as she snipped paper hearts with the dull scissors.

I didn't intend to say it, but I did, softly. "You know I will."

Chapter 34

❧

As the summer disappeared, a sadness settled over my wife like soot. Any attempt to remove it only succeeded in spreading it around, smearing it, making it uglier. I noticed the shabbiness of her car Goldie, her prized 1980 Firebird, a reminder of a happier time. Perhaps not happier. Different. She was single then and living alone, but she was healthy at least.

I took her car to an auto body shop, seeking a restored Goldie—a symbol that my wife, too, could be restored.

The auto man, an old Italian, eyed the car from a short distance. He squatted, scanned the solid body, the few spots of rust that were just beginning to form. "I look at this car, and I say you don't want a paint job. A car like this, you want done right. You want me to restore, no?"

I nodded my head. "I want it restored, yes."

"I restore, but it cost $2500."

"You restore it," I replied.

"You want gold?" he asked.

"That's her name. Goldie."

The car stayed in the shop for two weeks. When it was returned, it looked like a new car. Still gold, but a brilliant shimmering gold, with crisp black pin-stripes.

"Goldie's back!" my brother-in-law exclaimed. He remembered a few years back when the brakes were shot and we had talked of tossing her. He ran his hand across the smooth surface of the hood. "Great job."

My wife hobbled out with the help of her walker to view her car. She frowned. "You shouldn't waste your money on me," she sighed. "I'll never drive again." She climbed down from the porch and stepped a bit closer as I stood beside the car smiling.

"Then you can just look at her," I suggested. "Or I'll take you for a ride in her."

She stared at the new finish for a brief moment, then turned toward the porch stairs.

"You don't like it?" I asked.

"I like it," she answered. "You just shouldn't be wasting money on me.

I did no more projects. I had followed the house painting with a bit of stone masonry. From winter through the summer, I had renovated the kitchen, dabbing on the last stroke of paint just before my wife's accident. It had been a lovely kitchen, but it was modern, not Victorian. I added a tin ceiling, some granite counters, wallpaper, a little white paint, and it was transformed into something that fit the style of the rest of the house.

Outside we had planted roses, repaired fences—there was always something. Now there was merely fatigue.

Once the kitchen was done, I had planned to redo the bathroom, to scrap the modern fixtures—the green tub and the pink-gray tile, the mirror wall. An old bear claw tub stood against a side of the garden shed, salvaged from a nearby house where the owners were headed in the opposite direction as us—modernizing. The fall leaves beckoned. I opened the shed door and stared at the tub. It would have to wait, I thought as I grabbed the rake.

Winter came early.

Each morning, I followed the same path into the city, took the same route to the train station, sat in the same seat. I sat in that seat so often that the conductor expected to find me there, and when I wasn't there, if I had taken a different seat, he would look anxiously out the window, wondering if perhaps I had missed my train, expecting to see me running across the poorly plowed parking lot in futile pursuit of the departing train.

From the train station, heading toward the office, I walked the same sidewalk, bought the same breakfast from the same coffee shop—medium black coffee and a low-fat cranberry muffin—and waited patiently for the same walk lights.

Even before leaving the house, my routine remained fixed. I shaved, took a pill, brushed my teeth, showered, made the bed. Downstairs, into the basement to put in one load of laundry—never two—after moving the previous day's load into the dryer. Unload the dishwasher, open the blinds, make the coffee.

It was through this fixed routine that I felt secure, felt that if I could predict the first hour of the day, then the rest of the day was known, that I somehow controlled it. And if the day was known, then the week followed, and so forth and so on.

When she got ill again—the fourth time—this security failed me. In little ways. I'd forget to take my pill and have to go back upstairs. The blinds would be left down and the house plants would suffer for it. The city became strange, a dark unfamiliar place full of unknown dangers: ice falling from buildings toward my skull with evil intent; amateur bank robbers foiled in their attempts by vigilant cops, catching me in the cross fire. A tow truck lifting a car, its taut cable threatening to snap loose and decapitate me as I walked by.

I'd sit at my desk, strum my fingers across the mahogany surface, make random indentations on my mouse pad with a fingernail. I was safely at work, but was our daughter all right? I'd become haunted by the nagging feeling that danger lurked everywhere: a pervert hiding among the bushes as she walked to school accompanied only by her imagination and her invisible sisters; germs festering on the unwashed bathroom drinking cup, developing into new strains, virulent forms never seen before, preparing to strike her down with unimaginable swiftness; spiders in the far corner of her room, toxic venom, waiting to drop on the unsuspecting child.

And then there was my wife. Should I call home just to hear her voice?

I cursed my loss—the loss of serenity, the inability to move forward without fear. But then I thought of her. My enemies were not real, just phantoms occupying dormant regions of my brain. My dangers were of my own making, but hers were real.

I did call her. "Hi."

"Hi," she said. "Not busy today?"

"How is everything?"

"Fine," she replied.

Even through the distortion of a telephone, I loved her voice.

I could hear my daughter in the background. Safe. "Victoria, Helmut, Chocolate, Chadwick, Jessica, Priscilla." She was calling out the names of our stuffed bears, my wife's bears. My wife had her recite them on days when I wasn't there so my daughter would know the bear's names and they wouldn't become forgotten.

"You missed Thadeus," I heard my wife say.

"Thadeus," the little girl responded.

Christmas approached. She had not regained her strength and only climbed the stairs on weekends to use the shower. And I slept upstairs, alone. I could have moved a bed downstairs and joined her, but that would have been admitting defeat. "Soon you'll be strong enough to climb the stairs to our bedroom," I promised her.

She smiled and said nothing.

"I could have them install one of those mechanical stair-climbing chairs, if you want."

"It would be a waste of money," she replied. "Soon I'll be dead and you'll be free."

No. Then I'll be lost.

She heard me as I returned home. "How was work?" she called.

I threw a wad of Kleenex into the trash disposal, then set my briefcase on the kitchen counter and strolled casually into the parlor.

She looked at me and her smile turned sad. "What's wrong?" she asked.

Our daughter came in carrying a Styrofoam ball. It was

covered with rustic red stars cut from construction paper by a child's dull scissors, each star held tenuously in place by a wad of Scotch tape. "I made you a Christmas ornament," she announced. She held it up in front of her mother's eyes.

"It's lovely," she replied.

I took the ornament and walked over to the flashing tree.

"Next to the clown," my wife said.

Yes, of course. Next to the clown. The clown ornament handmade somewhere in eastern Europe, bought in Halifax the day before her leg broke. I had hung it cautiously, not wanting it to break. I would wrap it carefully after Christmas; it would be the first thing off the tree. I would wrap it carefully in tissue paper, then slide it back into its original package. I would cover the package with bubble wrap and place it last in the box of ornaments, on top where it wouldn't break.

There were many things I couldn't stop from breaking in this world, but I would see that the glass clown from Halifax never broke.

I hung the Styrofoam ornament next to the glass clown. It was our favorite area of the tree, decorated with those special ornaments. Ornaments whose histories we would always know. Ornaments whose histories our child would know. The Styrofoam ornament would not survive past this Christmas— the stars were already beginning to drop, the Scotch tape unable to hold on to Styrofoam. But for this Christmas, that was where it belonged, with the special ornaments.

"It's beautiful, sweetheart." She squeezed our daughter's face gently between her palms. "Now go play in the living room. Mommy wants to talk to Daddy."

I sat on the edge of her bed and took her hand.

She looked up at my face. "What's wrong?" she asked again.

"Nothing," I replied softly.

"You've been crying," she said.

I felt my face, but I could feel no tears.

"Your face is streaked," she explained.

"I was writing," I replied. "I was writing and it made me cry."

"On the train?" she asked.

"Yes," I replied. "I was writing on the train, and I cried in front of everybody, but I didn't care."

"You were writing about us?"

She knew that I was, but she asked it anyway.

I nodded. "Yes."

"I'd like to read it, but I've cried enough already."

"You don't want to read it," I sighed. "It will make you sad. I'll write something happy just for you. A private story that no one else can read."

"You're sweet," she replied, and she squeezed my hand. "I wish we had met sooner. Then we could have had a few good years together."

"They have been good," I replied. "They've been bad, but they've been good, too, being with you."

"Does your story have a happy ending?" she asked.

"It made me cry."

"There are many ways to cry," she sighed. "I know. I've cried them all."

"It's a sad ending, but it's happy, too."

"I'd like you to read it to me. Just the happy parts."

"But the happy parts are happy because of the sad parts," I explained. "They wouldn't be happy without the sad parts."

She smiled, knowing what I meant.

Our daughter returned carrying a second ornament. She was cheerful. She smiled as she held up her creation, made from the remnants of the construction paper—a rustic red globe taped together and garnished with scraps of tinsel she had salvaged from the floor. "I made one for Dada, too." She looked at my face, and her smile turned into a frown. "Why is Dada crying?"

I hadn't realized that I was.

"He's not crying, Honey," my wife replied. "It's just his allergies."

"Oh." She smiled again, and held the ornament up for us to see. "I was going to put stars on this one, but I ran out of tape!"

The three of us laughed. She had run out of tape. Of course she had. The ornament was covered with it, strips and strips of tape holding the hundred little pieces of paper together.

"Well, I see where it all went." I chuckled.

"There's more tape in Daddy's room," my wife told her, and our little girl ran happily out of the room and up the back staircase to find it.

We listened to her footsteps on the floor above and heard the scrape of a chair as she slid it toward my desk where the tape was kept.

I kissed my wife's hand. "You've done a fine job raising her." She smiled back.

"This house. . . ." She glanced around at the ceiling and over at the walls. I had never changed the wallpaper. We had planned to, but I never found the time. "It makes me feel like we were together once before."

I walked over to the metal IV pole and checked the clear plastic bags that hung from it, watching the clear liquid drip from the tube into the reservoir. "We've always been together," I replied. "For centuries."

"Could we try one more time after this?" she asked. "But we'll meet when we're younger this next time."

"Sure. I'll wait for you."

She smiled, happy that even now I wouldn't let my guard down and still insisted that she would be the one to outlive me. "But how will you know me?"

I returned to the edge of her bed and took her hand in mine. "I'll know you," I promised. "Just as I always have."

She squeezed my hand tighter. "If only it could be."

"It will be because we love each other."

She began to cry.

"Don't cry," I whispered.

"Then say something to make me happy," she begged.

Say it.

I kissed her, then looked into her eyes, trying to gather in mine all the determination and strength I had learned over the past six years.

Say it.

I looked into her face. The lights of the Christmas tree blinked their reds and blues and greens across the white quilt that lay over my wife's legs. Color flashed on the walls and across the high polish of the yellow pine floors, but only the green lights seemed to reflect on her face now.

Say it.

"You'll live to be a hundred." I kissed her. Her eyes looked up at me, the same eyes I had married centuries before. Then I whispered in her ear, "And I'll love you forever."

Chapter 35

✣

S HE THOUGHT I was driving too fast, a minor little event in a long string of little events that made me worry. "Speed limit's forty," she pointed out.

"I'm going thirty-five," I replied.

"It seems faster than that."

We were going to visit her oncologist. We had been going to her oncologist for six years, and it was the first time she complained about my speed.

At first I thought she was losing her battle. After six years, the cancer had won. She was fading slowly; she no longer cooked, she slept for long periods. I ordered takeout each night—she would carefully select an item from our collection of menus. Then one night, she didn't care.

"Order me anything," she sighed. "I'll eat it."

She had never done that before. She was always very specific, asking whether the ribs came with mashed potatoes or fries, not risking the crab meat if she suspected it was whitefish in disguise. It worried me. There was something strange going on inside my wife, something beyond breast cancer.

So much had happened to her that I allowed myself to think that, yes, perhaps she was dying. Four, five rounds of chemotherapy. A bone marrow transplant. Radiation—ten, twelve rounds of ten visits each. Hormone treatments—Tamoxifen, Luprilide, Arimidex. Finally male hormones—testosterone. She was going to quit if she sprouted a mustache.

"A mustache is okay," I replied. "But if you sprout a penis, we'll have to talk this treatment plan over."

We laughed. We laughed a lot. Sometimes all you can do is laugh. She fell into a large flower pot in the kitchen and remained stuck in it for forty-five minutes. Her mother came by and found her there. I came home from work and saw the flattened flowers. My wife told me what had happened.

"Did the flower pot break your fall, or did it hurt?" I asked. "Because I can either put more flower pots around if you think it helped, or I can get rid of them if it hurt."

We laughed again.

She ordered Chinese food off the wrong side of the menu, then she fell again, so I called her oncologist and said I thought the cancer had spread to her brain. He ordered a CAT scan. The results showed a large tumor filling the left side of her head.

"It's in a good place, though," he explained. "It's between the skull and the brain lining. We can get it out."

I didn't argue with him. I knew what he meant, but his phrasing was poor. It was not in a good place. A good place for a tumor would have been on the trunk of an old elm tree, not on someone's brain.

৳৯

Quietly, I entered my wife's hospital room and saw her swollen face. I couldn't help asking myself, "Is it worth all this?"

"It's the cortisone," she told me. "It's made my face puffy."

"That's weird," I said. "They give you the cortisone to reduce swelling in your brain, but then it makes your face swell up."

"Don't try to understand it," she sighed wearily. "It's modern medicine." She shifted her bloated legs, looking for that one spot where they would be comfortable, if only for a few minutes. "I don't look in the mirror anymore," she said. "I don't even want to think of what I must look like."

She was still in there somewhere, hidden behind that battered, puffy face. There was a bright red and purple bulge beneath her right eye; she said it was from where they took a bone sample. I didn't ask for details—I imagined it had something to do with plucking bone chips out through her eye socket. Her left cheek was still bruised from when she fell, her last fall, the one that made me call her doctor and report that something was not right.

Her head was shaven. The surgeon didn't want to get to her brain through her forehead—that would have left a visible scar. Above the hairline, the scar would not show. There was a hose coming out of her neck. I pointed to it. "They give me my medicine through that," she explained as she sipped water through a straw.

I nodded sullenly.

My wife stopped sipping her water. "I think I only have to stay three more days," she reported. "They won't put my bone back until next week, though."

A piece of her skull was in a freezer somewhere in the bowels of the hospital, waiting for the swelling in her brain to go down. She would have to go home with a hole in her head. The skin was back in place, but it would bulge out later when the radiation treatments caused her brain to swell even further. She would look as if a baseball had hit her on the head.

Later she would return so the surgeon could put the bone back in. I worried that they wouldn't find it then—hospitals were always losing things. Once they lost my entire wife, so what chance did one little bone fragment stand? I would have felt better if they had let me leave the hospital with the piece of skull tucked safely in my breast pocket.

"You're snapping back," I exclaimed, trying to sound cheerful.

"Yeah, your little elastic band," she sighed.

After fighting for six years now, she was still my little elastic band, but she was a band of steel, too.

She pulled the straw from her lips and set the glass of water on the hospital table. "They still don't know if it's benign or malignant." She stretched her hands out toward me. She wanted to take a walk. She wanted to take a walk with her husband and not with a nurse. She hadn't been able to walk without assistance since her leg broke the prior summer.

I reached out, took her hands, and pulled her gently from her bed. "The surgeon said it really doesn't matter whether it's benign or not. He got it all out." I pushed her walker closer to the bed. "He also said he doesn't operate unless the patient is expected to live at least another six months."

She grabbed the handles of the walker and stood up. "Then I've got at least six months."

"Your oncologist said he thinks you have years left. He said you're an incredible woman."

She smiled. Her puffy face looked like a jack-o-lantern.

She was an incredible woman.

We walked slowly to the end of the hall, then back to her room. She liked having me there, to fluff pillows and water her flowers. They were tasks that the nurses or the aides would have done, but it meant more to her when it was done out of love.

"You'd better go home," she suggested, worried that our daughter would feel neglected.

"I suppose so." I looked once more at my wife's swollen face. I kissed her just below the oxygen hose protruding from her nostrils. What was it I asked? Was it all worth it?

I thought of our daughter waiting back home, planning the theme for her seventh birthday party. She had narrowed the choice down to royalty or animals. She was never supposed to know her mother.

Her mother was not supposed to survive past our daughter's first birthday, but she had lived to hear her say her first words and to see her lose her first tooth. She had seen her dressed as a firefly in her first dance recital. She had hobbled up the stairs of the aging grammar school and listened proudly as the teacher spoke of our daughter in glowing terms.

I thought of the time my wife and I held hands below the majestic Grand Tetons, before she was ill. I recalled the summer day we strolled through a meadow in Montana and ran in fear from bear poop, as if bear poop could hurt us. I thought sadly of what she had gone through since. She had changed. I had changed, too.

Had it been worth it? Whenever I looked at our daughter standing beside her mother's wheelchair, giving her a big hug— "I love you, Mommy"—doubt disappeared.

It had been worth the struggle.

But it wasn't fair.

Epilogue

I ALWAYS THOUGHT she would get better, right up until the very end. It was no more possible to think of the world without her than it was to think of the world without me.

She lay in bed, her lips crusted over with dried blood, asking me to move the trees out of her way. I suppose then she knew she was going somewhere; she needed a clear path. There was something there that we, the living, could not see.

"Yes, I'll move the trees," I replied softly.

She accepted her death long before I did.

"You can still get better," I told her. How many times had I said that? But she always smiled back at me as though I were a small child talking of Santa Claus.

"You're such a dreamer," she replied.

True. I was a dreamer. But any life worth living is built upon dreams. And even now, I take refuge in my dreams, sleeping in our silent house in our empty bed. I can dream then of her and me on a sandy beach, warm tropical waters, and the vibrant love of a young couple. We come alive once more; and I hate the morning light for dashing those dreams.

We were not a couple, though. Perhaps at first we were, but we grew quickly into a unit. Our hearts and minds joined as one, and we barely needed to speak. We were a silent pair walking hand-in-hand, pausing before the storefront to view the Christmas display. Secret smiles, sharing thoughts. Even that was stolen from us in the end.

"Is the Duchess coming for tea?" she asked, and I had no idea what she meant. Pain gripped my chest. She and I were breaking apart, and I felt the harsh anguish of our separation.

"Mommy scares me." Our daughter stood in a corner of the kitchen, her back pressed up against the wallpaper that my wife had so carefully selected. Was it last year? Yes, it was only last winter that she and I had redecorated the kitchen.

"Mommy's sick," I explained as I wrapped my hurting arms around the little girl. "The medicine's making her talk funny."

"She won't get better this time."

"No," I replied calmly.

"Someone get me a mustache," my wife called, and my pain increased.

I squeezed my daughter tighter in my arms and kissed her hair. "But you must still love her."

"I do, Dada," she replied. "It's just she scares me."

I abandoned my job and stayed home, searching for ways to bring joy to a woman who had seen so little joy lately. I found she liked me to scratch her back, along the band of scars left by a recent outbreak of shingles. I could tell she liked it by the way she moaned. Not pain, but pleasure.

"What do you call that?" she asked vaguely.

"What I'm doing?"

"Yes," she replied, her head sunken deep within her pillow.

"Scratching."

"Overacting?"

Close enough.

I adjusted her head, and saw another blood stain upon the pillowcase, the blood hers, of course, but the source unknown. We developed our own language, one that constantly changed as the cancer and the morphine fought each other for control of her brain.

I needed to touch her. Always. "You want me to overact?"

She opened her eyes briefly and stared at me. "No." She wet her cracked lips with her dry tongue. "Could you make my feet go away, though?"

"Sure," I replied. Our language had changed once more. I ran my fingers up and down her spine.

"Don't stop," she moaned.

"Never," I replied softly.

I took refuge in the kitchen, escaping the insanity our lives had become. But there was no escape. I washed the paring knife, and as I stared down at it, the vivid memory of the loving wife she had once been echoed through my mind.

You didn't put that knife in the dishwasher, did you?—a pet peeve of hers.

I wanted to hear her say that just once more. No, not once more. Forever.

I'm sorry, honey. I did.

The hot water will ruin it.

Yes, dear.

I wanted our old life back; even the life of the week before, when she could no longer walk and barely talked, but we could at least sit together in bed and watch the daytime talk shows—*My husband beats me, but I just can't leave him.*

I love my wife, but she just can't stay.

It wasn't to be, though.

Instead, she called deliriously, "It's lukewarm in the hot tub. Fetch me a rubber ducky!"

She haunted my thoughts. I mourned her passing even though she was still alive. I would look at her silent figure, so small now, unconscious on her sickbed, and I would recall the last time she had walked, moving ever so slowly among the stalls of the antique market, picking up ceramic bowls and feeling along their yellowed edges for chips. I followed behind, pushing her wheelchair. Our daughter sat on it, enjoying the free ride, but it was really there for my wife, waiting for her legs to give out. I was impatient then, wondering why my wife must pick up every object; but I knew now, she was touching life, past and present, absorbing it because she knew she had no future. I would gladly walk behind her again; I would not need patience because it would be such a pleasure, and our moments together would seem too fleeting.

How many weekends had we cruised the antique shops of Route 1? Fifty? A hundred? Yet to be able to do it just once more would still be priceless.

"We haven't been communicating well this week, have we?" My wife smiled, her teeth black and grotesque—the final outrage to her wasted body.

A bit of her had returned. One last spark of her precious life—of our precious life—glowing ever so faintly under the lights of the Christmas tree.

"No, we haven't," I agreed. I wanted to clean her teeth, remove the blood and make them white again, but I didn't know how. She couldn't spit, and I might drown her in toothpaste.

It was not just her teeth, though. There was so much of her I wanted to fix: her crumbling bones, the hole in her skull, the tumor in her brain, the scars upon her body. But I couldn't even clean her teeth.

I tried a bit of wet cheesecloth, but she thought I was feeding her and gripped it between her black teeth.

I sat in darkness for six nights, listening to her steady breath, little bits of our past flitting from her dreams, bringing a sad smile to my face as I recalled the moments she was dreaming of. Barbados, Hawaii.

"Grammy! Grammy! Quick! To the river's edge."

All the way back to her childhood, to a simpler, happier time.

"Put your raincoat on. You'll get wet."

"Watch out for crazies on the road."

"Make sure there's no bears in there."

Even in her delirium, she was thinking of my safety.

I sat in darkness until the morning light, and then I heard our daughter singing in the bathroom. I waited until she came downstairs, and I took her hand.

"I'll walk you to school today."

Together we stepped outside. Although it was not yet winter, the air was frigid. The night clouds had cleared, leaving only their faint memory on the eastern horizon.

I blinked in the harsh morning light. The sidewalks were crowded with children on their way to school. White clouds burst from the cold engines of our neighbors' cars. The drivers smiled and waved as they backed onto the street and headed to their jobs.

Turning, tears flooding my eyes, I viewed the rose bushes my wife had planted. A sad smile spread across my face as I scanned the house, the Queen Anne Victorian that she had chosen out of all the others. I felt our daughter's grip—"Come on, Dada. I got to get to school"—and I knew that my wife would never leave me.

But she would die, and that night she did. Quietly, at home where she wanted to be, her mother and sister joining me at her side. Her white lips moved ever so slowly—twice, like a small fish—and then she exhaled her final breath.

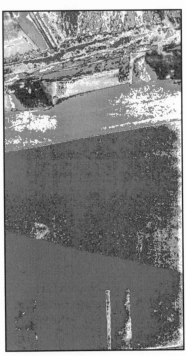

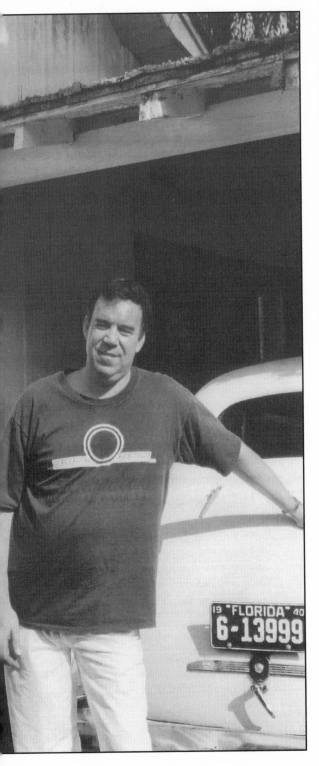

David Tillman lives in Massachusetts with his eight-year-old daughter and three bunnies. They are avid skiers, and will travel miles out of their way for a motel with a warm pool. Since his wife's death, Mr. Tillman has been striving for total ignorance of the world he now lives in alone—he reads novels, writes plays, short stories and memoirs, and is a systems consultant to Boston Investment firms.